SEXTROLOGY

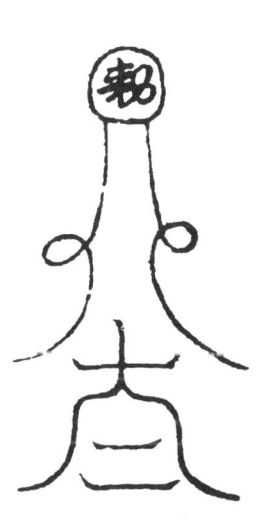

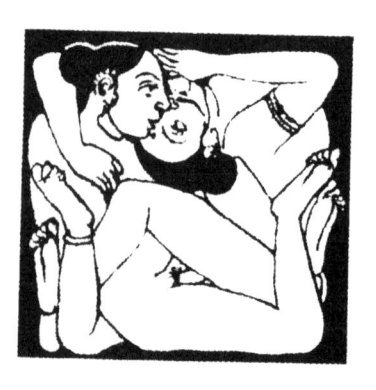

Edward B. Gould

SEXTROLOGY

Astrology for a great sex life

Astrolog Publishing House

Illustrations: Daniel Akerman

Astrolog Publishing House
P. O. Box 1123, Hod Hasharon 45111, Israel
Tel: 972-9-7412044
Fax: 972-9-7442714
E-Mail: info@astrolog.co.il
Astrolog Web Site: www.astrolog.co.il

Astrolog Publishing House © 2002

ISBN 965-494-143-0

All rights reserved. No part of this publication may be reproduced, stored in a retrieval system, or transmitted in any form or by any means, electronic, mechanical, photocopying, recording or otherwise, without the prior permission of the publisher.

Published by Astrolog Publishing House 2002

1 3 5 7 9 10 8 6 4 2

Contents

Introduction	9
Sex in the mirror of your house	15
Positions	19
Aries	65
Taurus	76
Gemini	87
Cancer	98
Leo	109
Virgo	119
Libra	130
Scorpio	140
Sagittarius	151
Capricorn	161
Aquarius	172
Pisces	182

In the following two pages, you can feast your eyes on the 36 positions that will be explained later on.

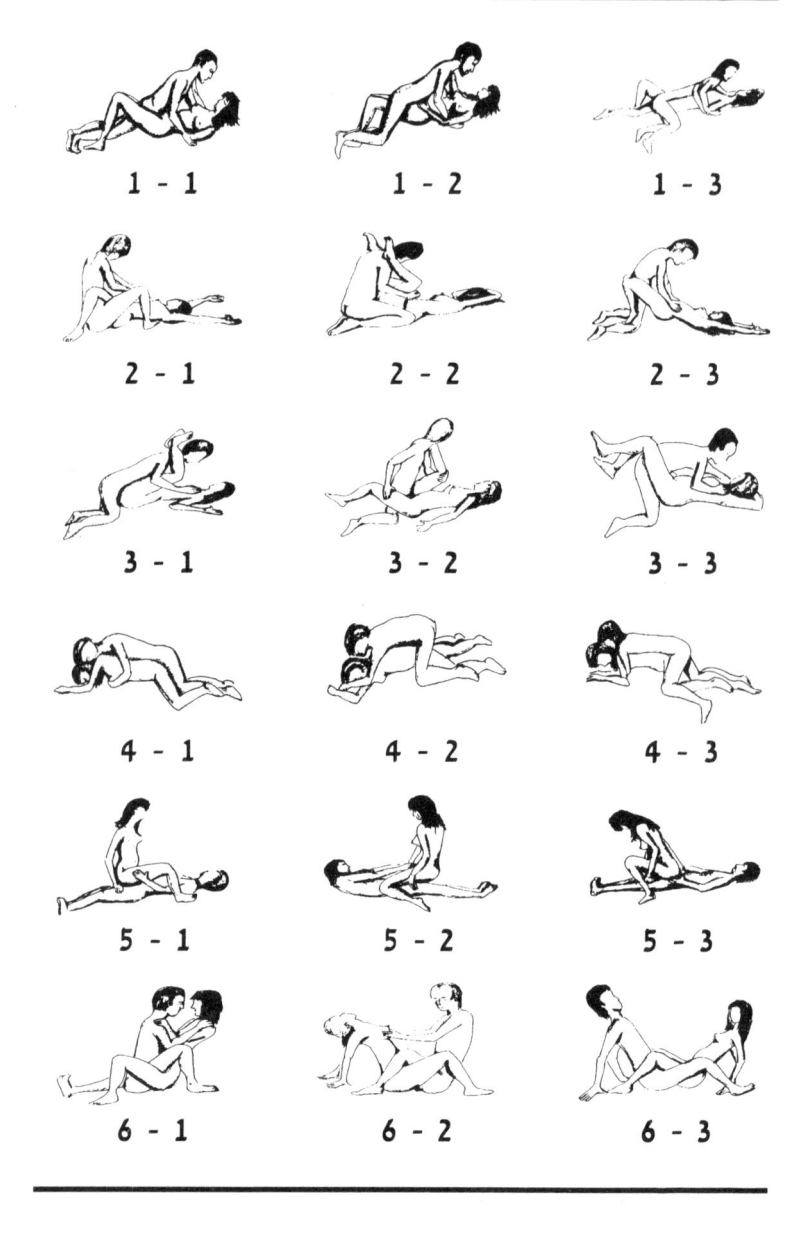

Positions

1 - 1   1 - 2   1 - 3

2 - 1   2 - 2   2 - 3

3 - 1   3 - 2   3 - 3

4 - 1   4 - 2   4 - 3

5 - 1   5 - 2   5 - 3

6 - 1   6 - 2   6 - 3

Positions

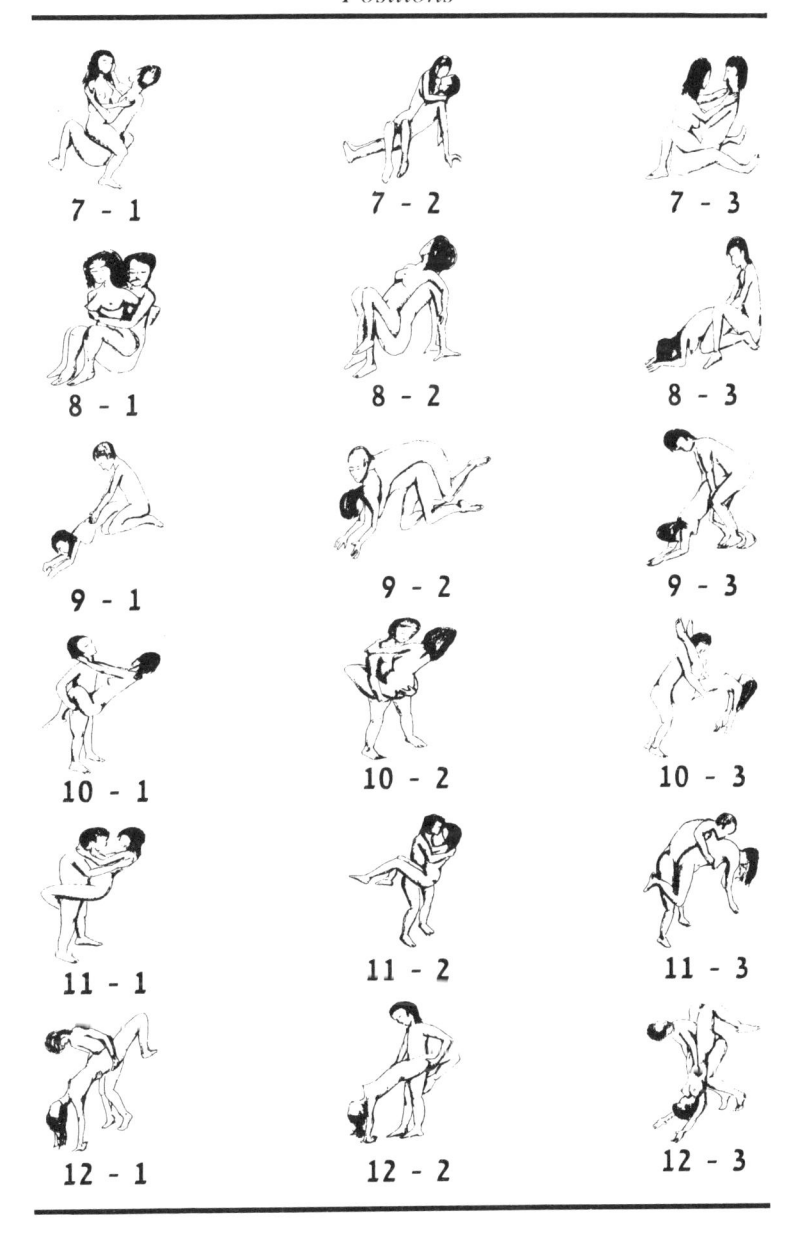

7 - 1

7 - 2

7 - 3

8 - 1

8 - 2

8 - 3

9 - 1

9 - 2

9 - 3

10 - 1

10 - 2

10 - 3

11 - 1

11 - 2

11 - 3

12 - 1

12 - 2

12 - 3

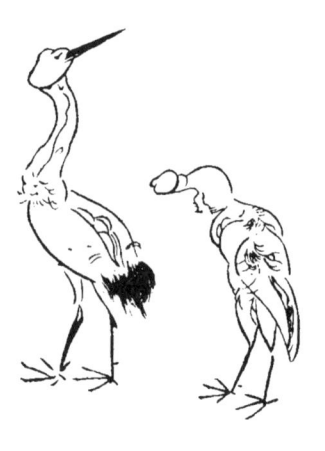

Introduction

As everyone knows, the most famous erotic writings in the world came from the East. The *Kama Sutra*, for instance, was written in India in the fifth century CE, as was the *Ananga Ranga*, or the *Kama Shustra*. In China, erotic manuals called the *Golden Lotus* were written, in addition to books such as *The Tao of Lovers*. In Japan, there were the splendid *Shunga* books. In the East, Islamic eroticism was expressed in *The Thousand and One Nights* and in the *Pleasure Garden*. Judaism, too, produced *The Song of Songs* as well as other fascinating erotic writings. All of these writings constituted an inseparable part of the Eastern astrologer's library. The reason for this was that the astrological advisor dealt with matters of sex, sexual compatibility, matches, and sexual problems as an indivisible part of his work.

What is the connection between these erotic scripts and astrology? Simple: all the erotic writings and astrological theories of the East, especially the one known today as Chinese astrology, were developed by the self-same sages.

Eastern astrologers learned a long time ago that people belonging to the different signs had different sexual natures. They also learned that men and women are endowed with genitals of different sizes and different erogenous zones, and have different preferences concerning sexual rhythm and positions, according to their particular sign.

The definition of the sexual character, or the sexual temperament, is important for every member of the particular sign... and is even more important for determining compatibility between the different signs. Don't forget... it takes two to tango!

An Eastern male who has received the correct tutelage is supposed to match his sexual activity to the sign of his partner. Concubines, or women who worked in "houses of pleasure" in the East, were also conversant with the required variations in their relations with the members of the various signs.

Only in recent years has the Eastern astrological sexual compatibility that is called sextrology reached the West. (Let us stress that we mean sexual compatibility in the physical sense, not just compatibility in the sense of "love" or matches, and so on.) In the East, we can still find detailed charts of scores of positions, and every couple can choose the position that suits its astrological signs. Moreover, sexual rhythm is also elaborated upon, and, of course, there is a great deal of information concerning topics such as size, staying power, and sexual temperament, which should be known before people engage in sex. This art is still in its infancy in the West.

The chapters of this book deal with the properties of the members of the various signs, describe the 144 possible couplings, and stress the type and content of the recommended sexual activity in each one of them. In addition, there is a detailed questionnaire that enables everyone to discover the extent of his/her compatibility with the "ideal" sextrological profile presented in the book.

Eastern sextrology consists of 36 basic positions, and not only do we elaborate upon these positions (with the help of illustrations), but we also discuss the compatibility between the members of a couple and the compatibility with members of different signs.

The chapters are divided according to the 12 signs of the Zodiac that are recognized in the West (after the dates of birth have been matched according to the accepted Eastern signs). Initially, we present the sexual characteristic for each sign, according to Western astrology. Only afterwards do we discuss the sexual temperament and properties of the various signs - men and women separately - and present the table of compatibility according to sextrology, including a selection of positions and rhythms preferred in every coupling.

Years ago, during one of my visits to Bangkok, the sex capital of Asia, I happened to go into one of the local "brothels." This book was born in the "brothel," and that chance visit changed my sex life dramatically for the better.

Perhaps I should preface my story with a few words.

This Eastern "brothel" deserves to be called a "house of pleasure." The girls who work in the place do not sell their bodies to men. Rather, they sell the art of love, which they learned in all its intricacies in special institutions that qualify girls, from a young age, to fulfill the requirements for working in the scores of houses of pleasure throughout Bangkok. (I should explain that my personal experience is with girls, but whatever is written in this book is also true of the boys who are available for the women who visit these places.)

As is customary, I was led into a small room upon my arrival, in the middle of which was a large sunken wooden tub for bathing.

Two girls undressed me, and after I had entered the warm bath, which smelled of roses, they washed my body with gentle hands. After drying my skin, I was dressed in a kimono - a thin silk robe - and entered the adjoining room. Physical cleanliness is a fundamental rule in sexual activity in the East.

"What is your date of birth?" one of the owners of the place - a woman of about 30 - asked me politely.

I was amazed. Up till then, I had been accustomed to questions of an entirely different nature. In houses of pleasure, they always wanted to know my preferences, what kind of sexual activity I was interested in, and so on. What did my date of birth have to do with my sexual proclivities?

I gave the exact date, hour, and place of my birth, and the woman approached an old man sitting in the corner, a pile of leather-bound books with yellowing pages in front of him. The old man took the note she had written, looked through the books, and began to make a list on a sheet of paper. Eventually, he wrote something on a bit of paper and handed it to the owner.

That was not the first time I had seen such lists. In the East, there are astrologers on every street corner. No Easterner will take any serious step concerning himself, his business, or his family, without consulting with an astrologer. But what was the connection between an enjoyable visit to a house of pleasure and astrology? I asked - and the answer astounded me!

"We want to match you with the best partner for your pleasures," answered the woman. "And the best way to do this is to match your signs of the Zodiac. The old man has matched your dominant sign to the sign of one of the girls, and I'm sure you'll have no regrets."

I found the subject intriguing. After several pleasurable hours with one of the girls - and believe me, there is nothing like these girls to drive a man insane with pleasure in bed - I went back to the old man and began to talk to him. This conversation sparked three years of research. Eastern astrology is influenced mainly by the wisdom of China and India, and the transition from it to the astrology that is predominant in the West is quite difficult. However, at the end of my research, after I had checked my conclusions, I devised a theory that I call the theory of sextrology.

This theory links the effect of the planets' radiation on every man and every woman's sexual behavior, preferences, abilities, and potential.

It is not just meant for finding mates and maximum compatibility. Sextrology can guide the man to the sexual positions that most suit him, guide the woman to reach heights of sexual release, spur on the "drooping" and "floppy" among the knights of the bedchamber, and make both men and women more aware of the stars' influence on their sex life. And this is doubly true when we examine the relationship between the members of a couple. This book must be read and studied with an open mind. The reader should not jump to hasty conclusions or ignore inconvenient warnings.

I hope that by using this book, the reader's sexual awareness and pleasures will be enhanced.

E.B.G.

According to Western Astrology

Sex in the mirror of your house

This brief chapter is presented for the convenience of readers who are conversant with conventional astrology and want to expand their knowledge of the sexual expression of the houses in the astrological map. Eastern astrology, too, attributes importance to the various houses of the birth map.

Like all astrology books, the study of sextrology also deals with the influence of the houses on the person's life.

As we know, there are twelve houses, and the significance of each one depends on a planet or the dominant sign for a particular person in the particular house. We have to find the dominant element for each house, and study the dozen houses in order to understand the characteristics of the person in various areas of sexual relations. Let's see what each of the houses characterizes:

The first house:
The structure of the personality and temperament of the person, as they are expressed at birth! This house is extremely important regarding the personal abilities that each person brings to the sexual encounter.

According to Western Astrology

The second house:

The ambitions and talents inherent in every person - the desire to do something and the ability to realize that desire. We sometimes forget that not everyone is eager for sexual activity... and the extent of a person's eagerness is determined in this house.

The third house:

The rational ability, and the important property of sexual expression. The ability to establish communication is the first step on the long road leading to the pleasures of sexual intercourse.

The fourth house:

This house focuses mainly on what the person received from his parents - in upbringing, attitude, and property. Its influence in the field of sexual relations occurs mainly in the development of deviations from what the person considers acceptable.

The fifth house:

The most important house! This house is linked to sex, and to every other activity that stimulates desire and enjoyment - in short, everything that is nice and is slightly "frowned upon."

According to Western Astrology

The sixth house:
This house dominates the person's health and physical fitness. As we know, the genitals are part of the body... and in fact, sound health of the entire body is a prerequisite for full enjoyment of active sexual relations.

The seventh house:
This house is mainly directed at the person's partner, and, after the fifth house, it is the most important one in determining sexual relations.

When it comes to sexual relations between men or between women, too, the influence of this house is of cardinal importance.

The eighth house:
This gloomy house deals mainly with death, or with the end of some kind of process. It exerts an influence on sexual impotence, and its influence is powerful during the change of life in both men and women.

The ninth house:
The person's world-view - puritanical or liberal, faithful or promiscuous, and other attitudes - is determined according to the influence of this house.

According to Western Astrology

The tenth house:
This house is linked to the person's work and career, and his dealings with superiors and subordinates, both at work and in interpersonal relationships. Master-slave relationships in sex are influenced by this house.

The eleventh house:
This is house of friendship, which influences the ties of companionship and friendship that the person establishes with those around him. Sexual relations are the development of these ties.

The twelfth house:
This house has been nicknamed "the prison." It influences the emotional impediments and inhibitions that affect the person. Sexual problems and inhibitions frequently stem from the influence of this house.

Positions

Let's get down to business. In the following pages, you will find the 36 favorite sexual positions. These are based on the 12 basic positions, each of which comes in three variations. The various characteristics of each position are described in detail.

The *Kama Sutra* and the *Ananga Ranga* are the two main sources from which the 36 basic positions in sextrology were derived.

In the East, these 36 positions are called "the pillars of marriage." They appear in writing for the first time in the eighth century CE in India. The 36 illustrations in the present book appeared in the first printed book containing the various positions - a book that was printed in Bombay in 1831.

At the end of this chapter, there are 4 tables:

A. **A table showing preference for positions according to signs of the Zodiac.**

B. **A table showing which signs favor which for positions.**

C. **A table showing the perfect sexual compatibilities for men (according to signs).**

D. **A table showing the perfect sexual compatibilities for women (according to signs).**

Sextrology

1. In the first basic position, the woman lies on her back, her shoulders, buttocks, and legs on the mattress, with the man lying on top of her, face to face, most of his weight on the woman. Their arms are free to move, and they can kiss each other. Parts of the woman's body are inaccessible to the man's hands (because they are squeezed against the mattress). What characterizes the first basic position is the fact that the legs of one or both of the couple are almost straight. Today, this is the basic position in every act of intercourse, and it is called the "missionary position" in the West. However, in the dawn of civilization, we hardly find this position, which requires a great deal of security and tranquillity. The basic position appears in the following variations, according to the position of the couple's legs:

1-1 When both of the man's legs are between the woman's spread legs.

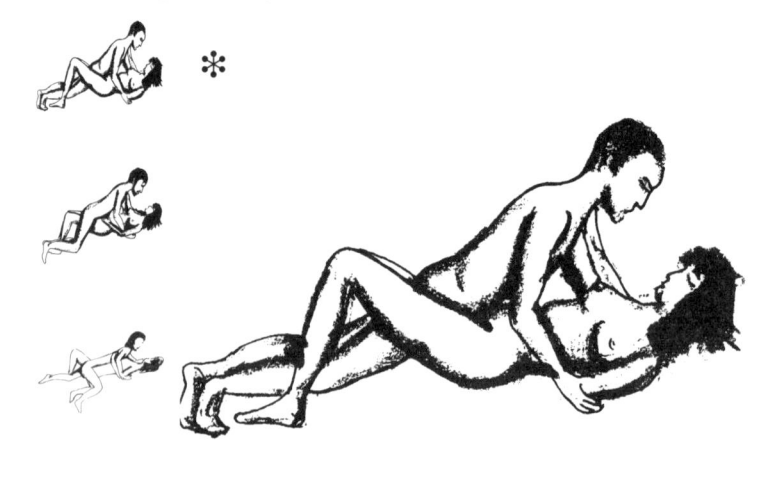

1-2 When both of the woman's legs are between the man's spread legs.

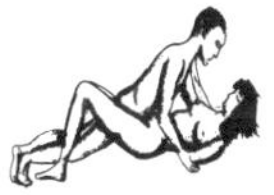

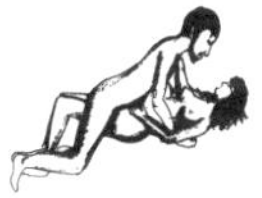 *

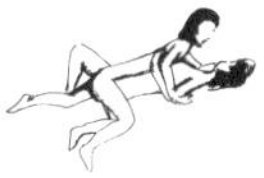

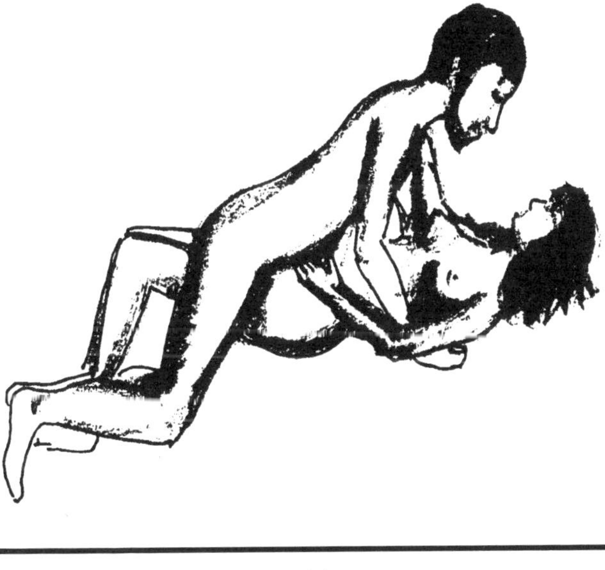

Sextrology

1-3 When one of the man's legs is between the woman's legs and his other leg is wrapped around the outer part of the woman's leg.

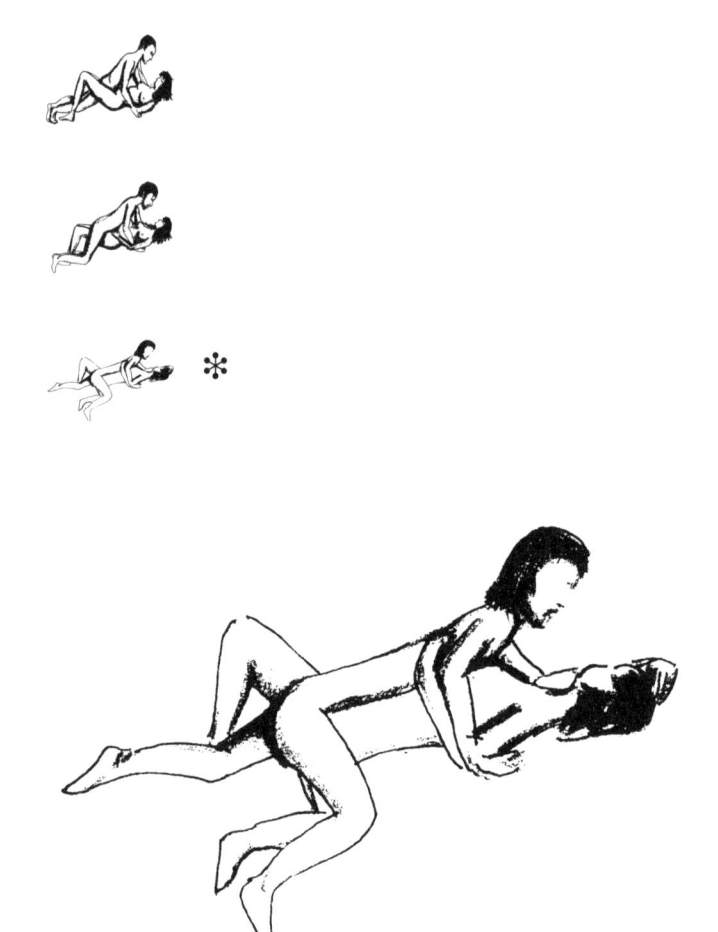

Sextrology

2. In the second basic position, the woman lies on her back, her arms supporting her body and her legs straight up in the air (even at right angles to her body) and supported on the man's shoulders or held in his hands, closed or spread. Her bottom touches the mattress but does not lie on it. The man is "behind" the woman's legs, holding or touching them, and his back is actually parallel to her legs. In this position, the woman and the man cannot kiss each other, and the extent to which they can caress each other depends on their pliancy. In this position, the man kneels or sits, and uses the woman's legs as a lever for moving his body. The basic position appears in the following variations, according to the positions of the man's pelvis and legs:

2-1 When the man is sitting on his bottom and his legs are bent at the woman's sides (his feet are parallel to his bottom).

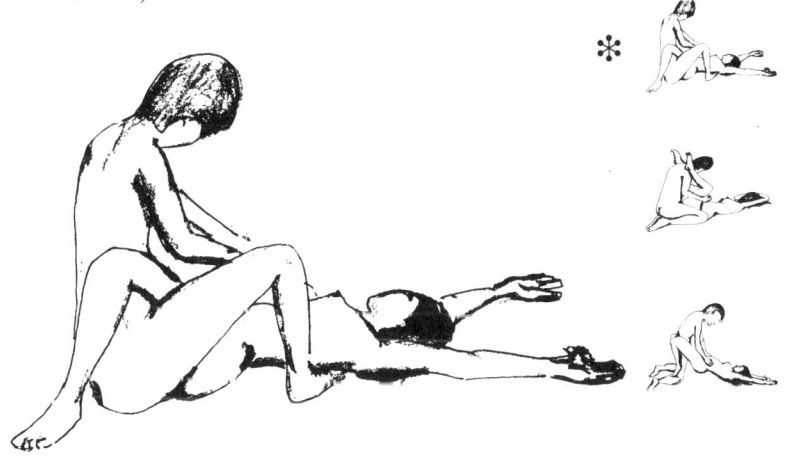

23

Sextrology

2-2 When the man kneels, his thighs resting on his calves and his bottom "sitting" on his heels.

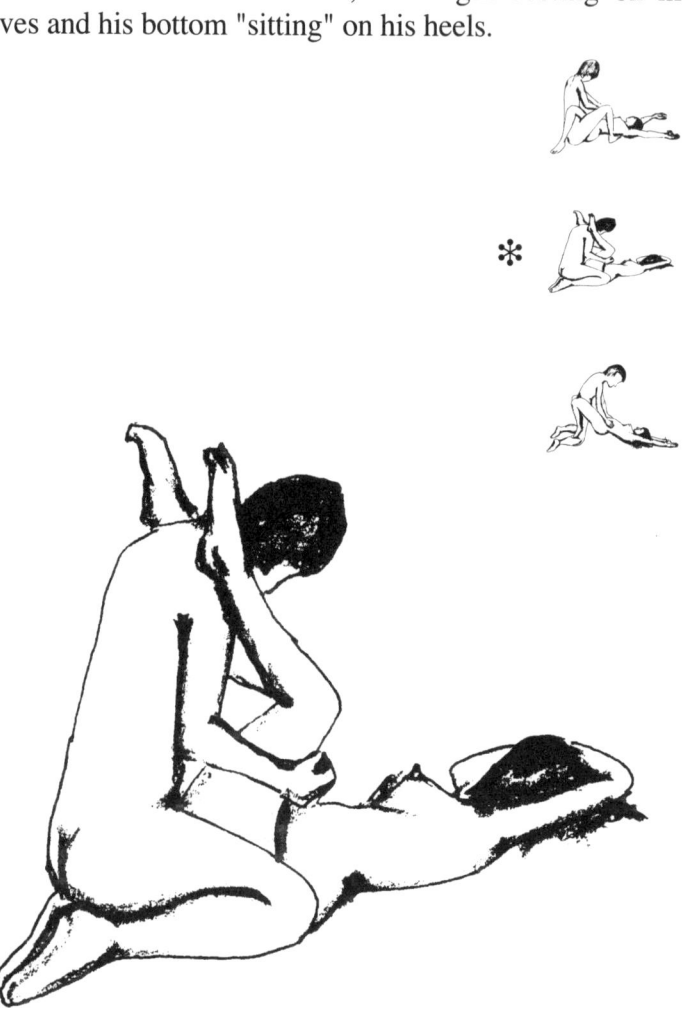

Sextrology

2-3 When the man kneels, his thighs in a straight line with his back (his knees form right angles) and the woman's bottom is lifted up and leans on the man's body.

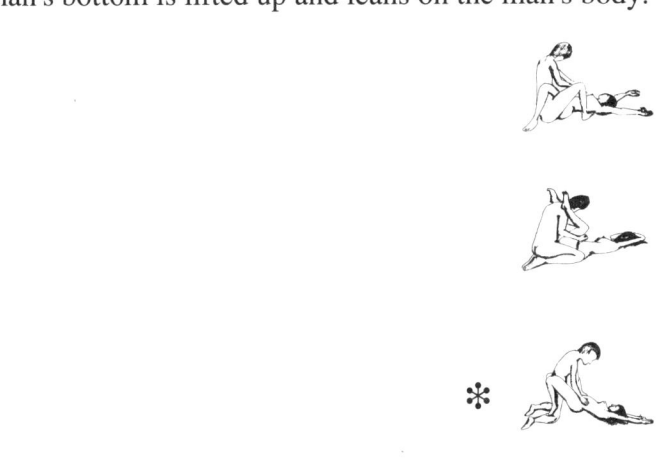

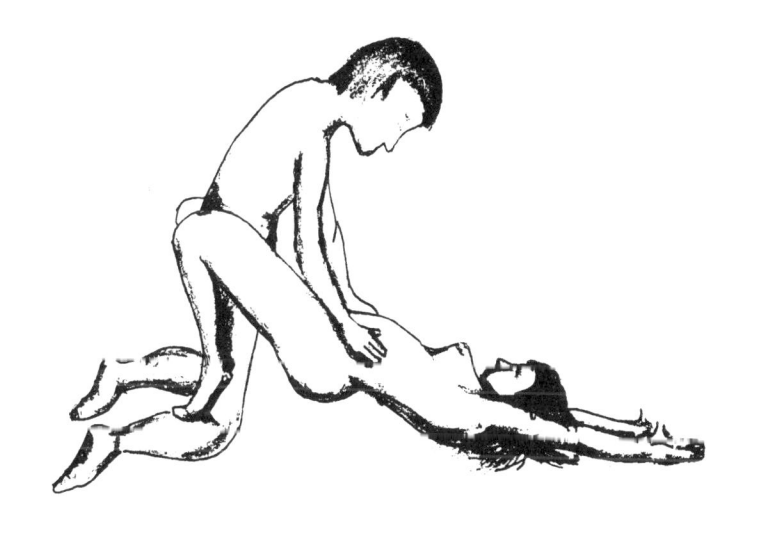

Sextrology

3. In the third basic position, the woman lies on her back, her arms supporting her body, as in the second basic position. The difference is that here, her legs are bent. The man is between her legs, kneeling and holding her legs. His hands are not free to caress the woman since they are leaning on her legs or holding them all the time. The position of the woman's legs here determines the variations in the basic position.

3-1 When both of the woman's legs are bent, spread, and pushed toward her head, so that her knees press onto her breasts.

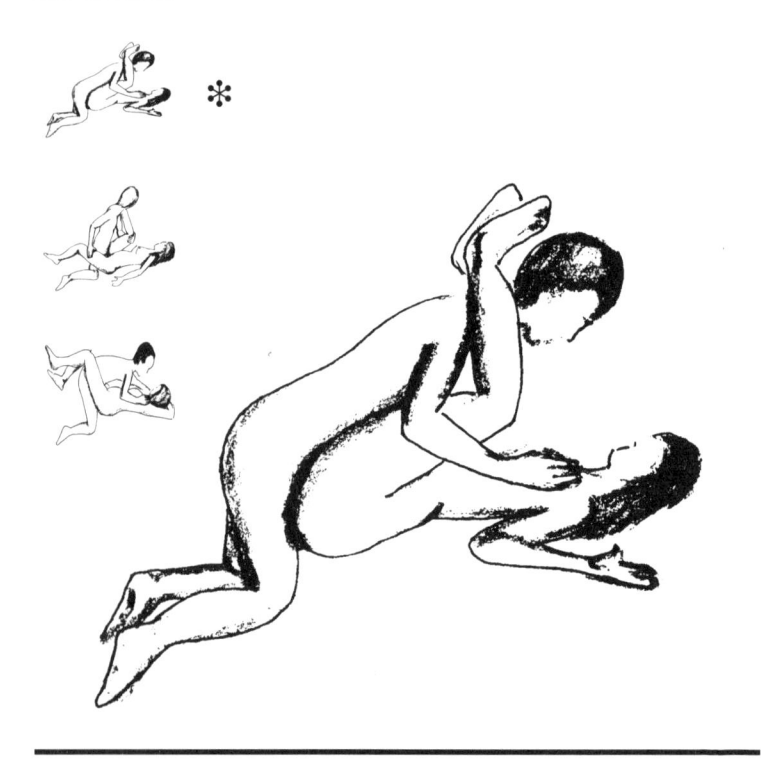

Sextrology

3-2 When one of the woman's legs is bent, spread, and pushed toward her head, while the other leg is bent and held on the man's hip or in his armpit.

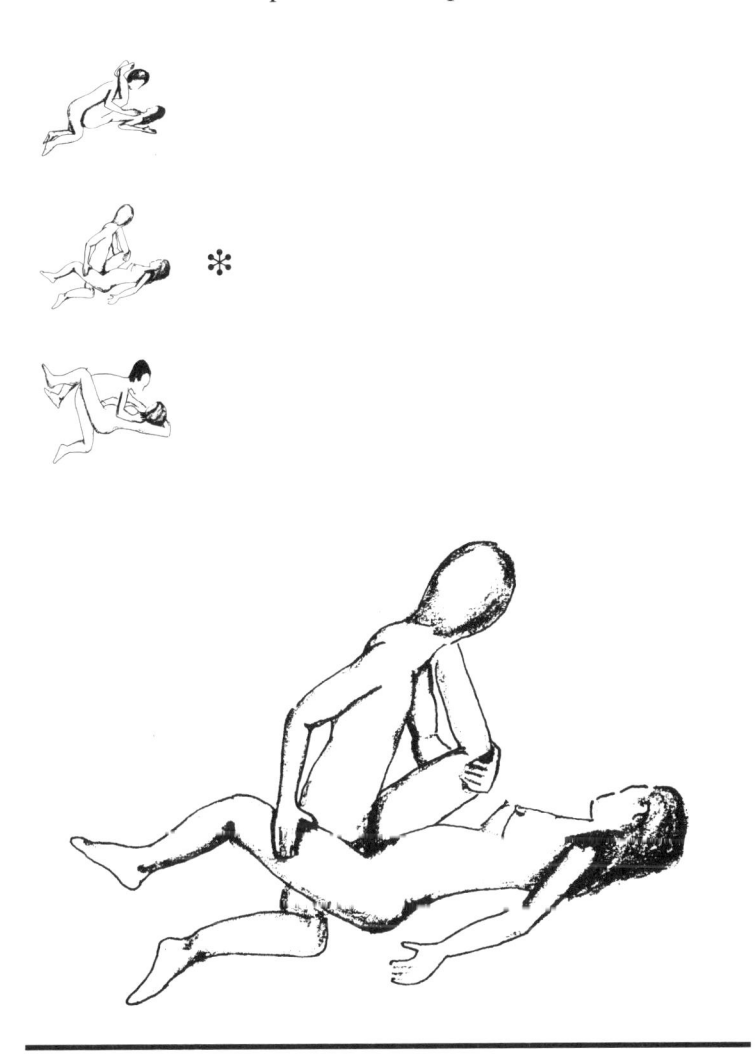

Sextrology

3-3 When both of the woman's legs are bent, spread, and held against the man's hips (on each side of his body) or in his armpits.

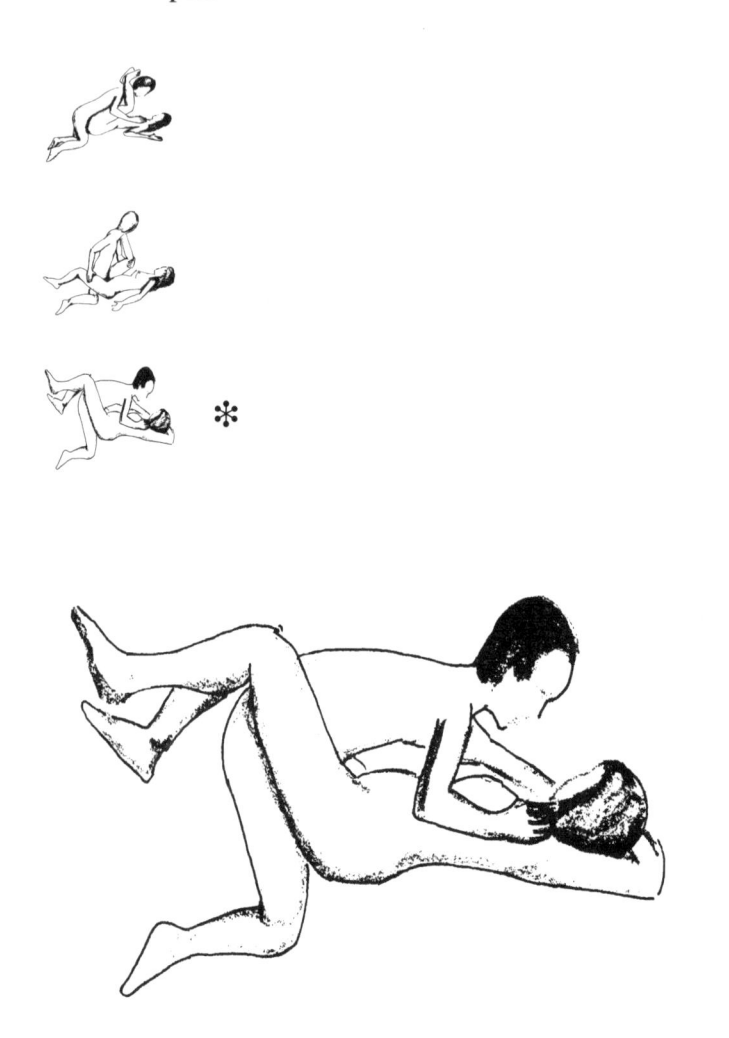

✜

Sextrology

4. In the fourth basic position, the woman lies on her stomach on the mattress, her face, abdomen and legs against the mattress, and the man lies on her back, his head above hers, his weight supported by her body and his knees. In this position, the man can use his hands and mouth, but the woman's ability to move is limited. The variations in this basic position are determined by the positions of both of their legs, as in the first basic position.

4-1 When the woman's legs are spread, and the man's legs are between hers.

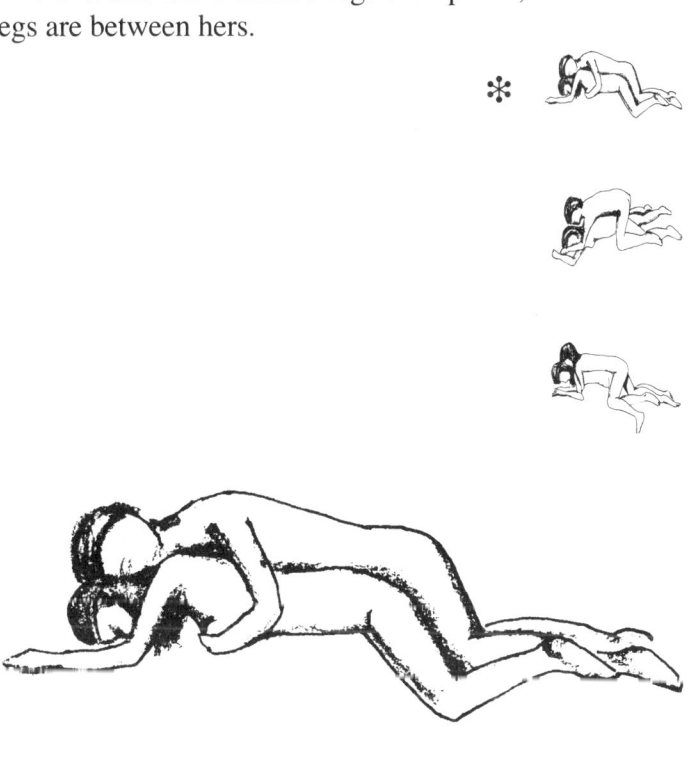

Sextrology

4-2 When the man's legs are spread, and the woman's legs are between his.

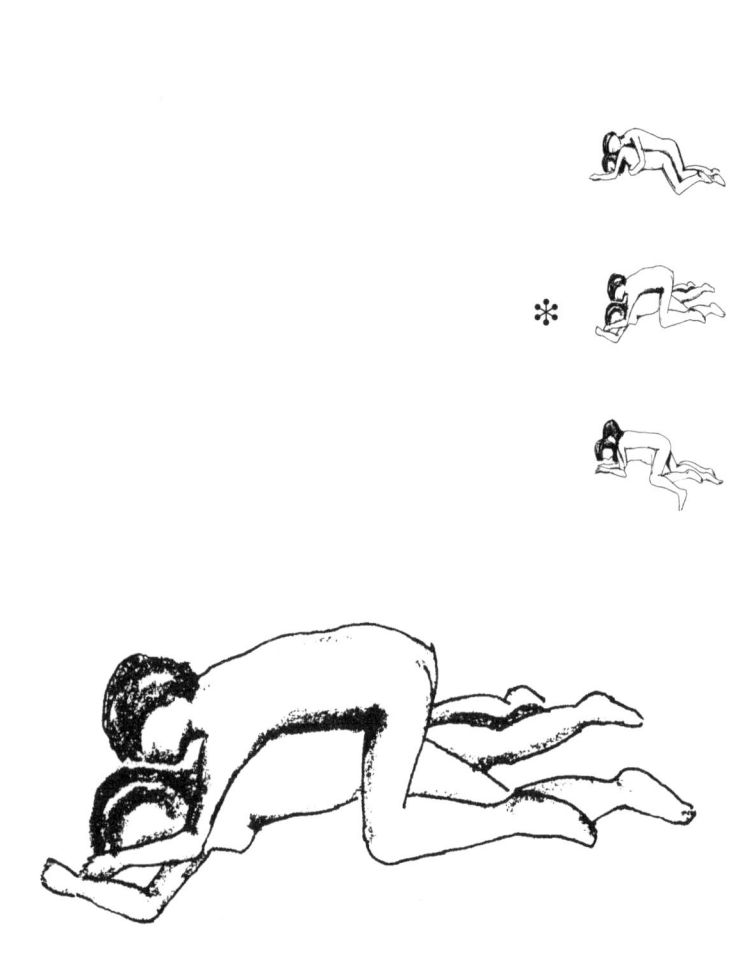

Sextrology

4-3 When one of the man's legs is between the woman's legs, and his other leg is wrapped around one of her legs.

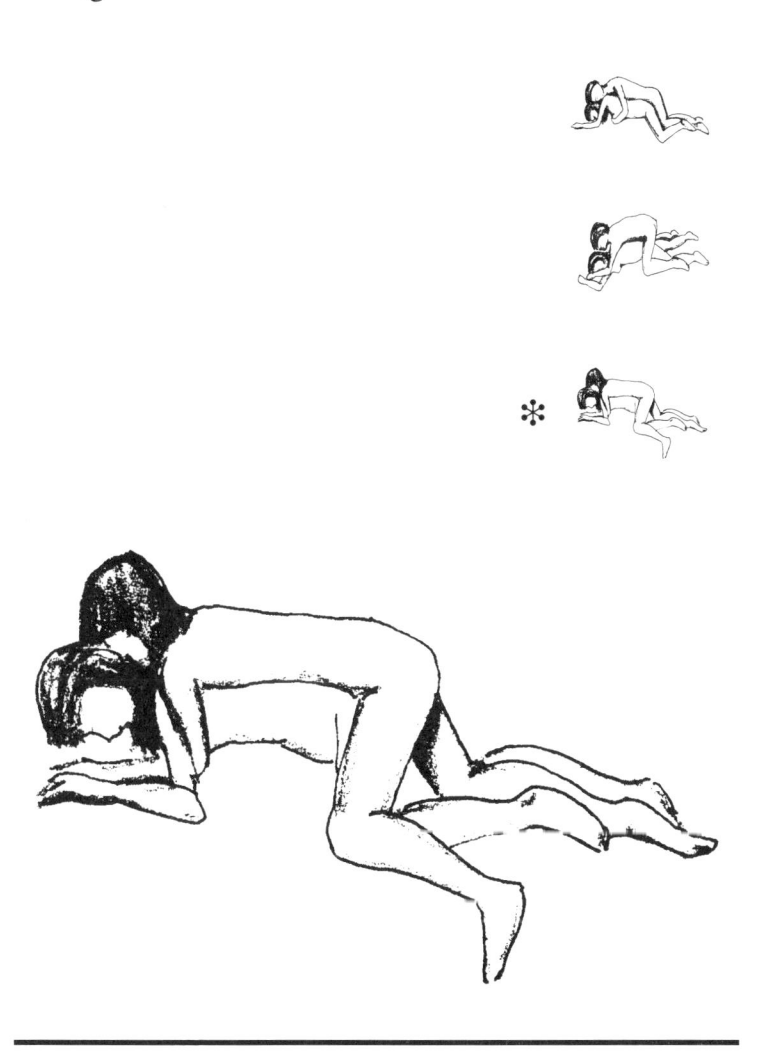

Sextrology

5. In the fifth basic position, the man lies on his back, his shoulders, bottom and legs on the mattress, with the woman on his body. She hardly touches the mattress. This position enables the woman to control the rate of intercourse (and this is exactly why in many cultures, this position is considered to be scandalous, since the woman is the one who does the work). It is mainly suitable in cases in which the man is tired and does not have a full erection, and in cases when their genitals are not compatible in size. (It is also good in cases of advanced pregnancy.) The sitting position of the woman determines the variations on this basic position:

5-1 When the woman sits facing the man, her legs straight out in front of her on either side of his head (her heels on his shoulders) and she supports her body with her arms, her hands on his thighs.

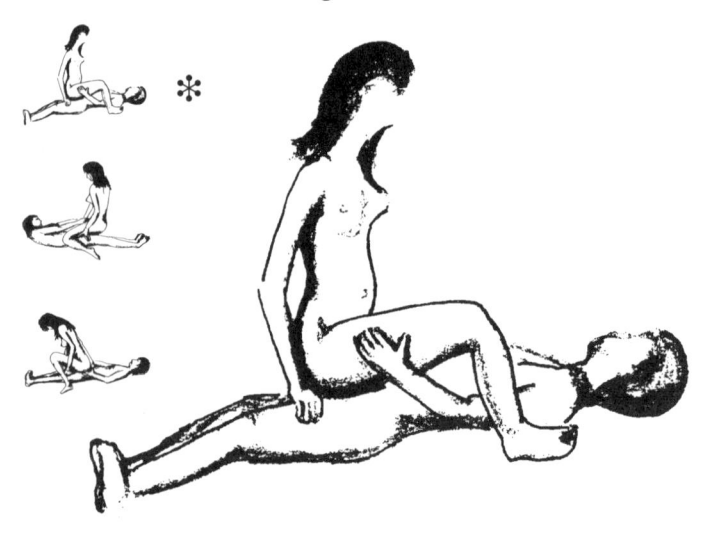

Sextrology

5-2 When the woman sits facing the man, her legs bent on either side of his abdomen (or crossed in lotus or cross-legged position), her hands leaning on his abdomen and supporting her body.

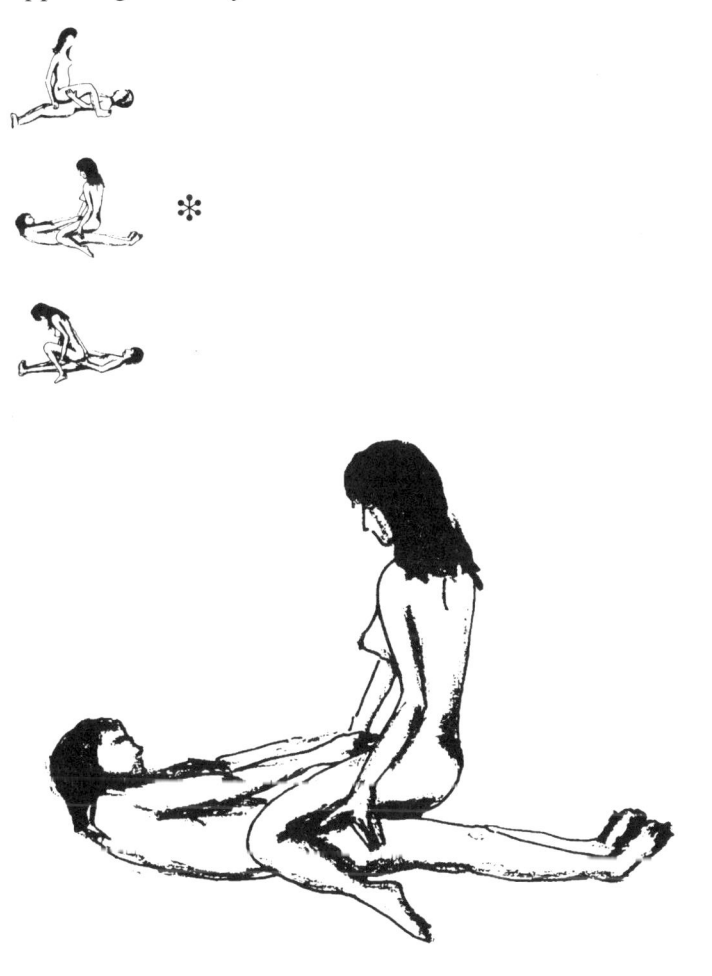

Sextrology

5-3 When the woman sits facing the man's feet (her back to his face), her legs bent on either side of him and her hands leaning on his legs in order to support her body.

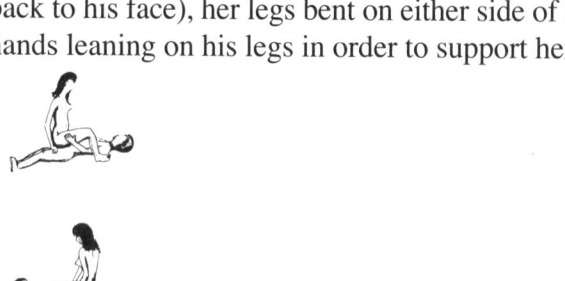

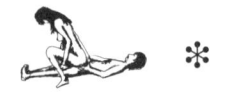

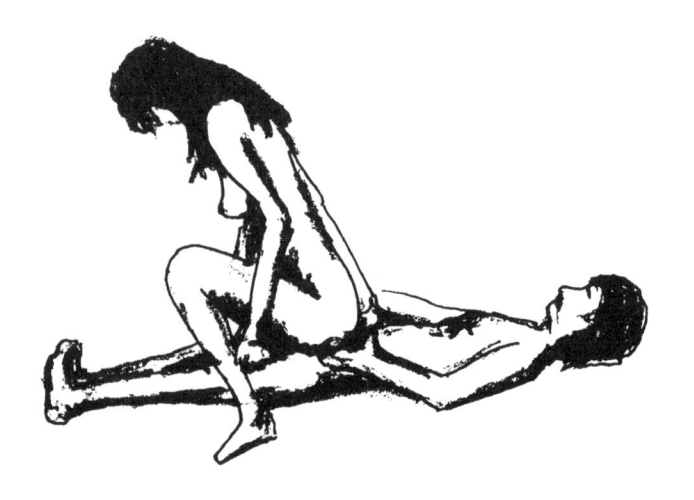

Sextrology

6. In the sixth basic position, both partners sit facing each other. This position enables both of them to kiss and use their hands for caressing each other. It is described in the Hindi culture as "tree-trunks touching" - in order to achieve sexual contact, they must push their pelvises together. The "roots," that is, their legs, can be in any position - straight, bent - but not on top of one another. Their arms support their partner and at the same time serve as a lever and anchor for equilibrium. In this position, the couple's pliancy and physical fitness are important. The position of the "branches," that is, the upper part of their bodies, determines the variations here:

6-1 When their backs are upright and they are close to each other, stomach to stomach and chest to chest.

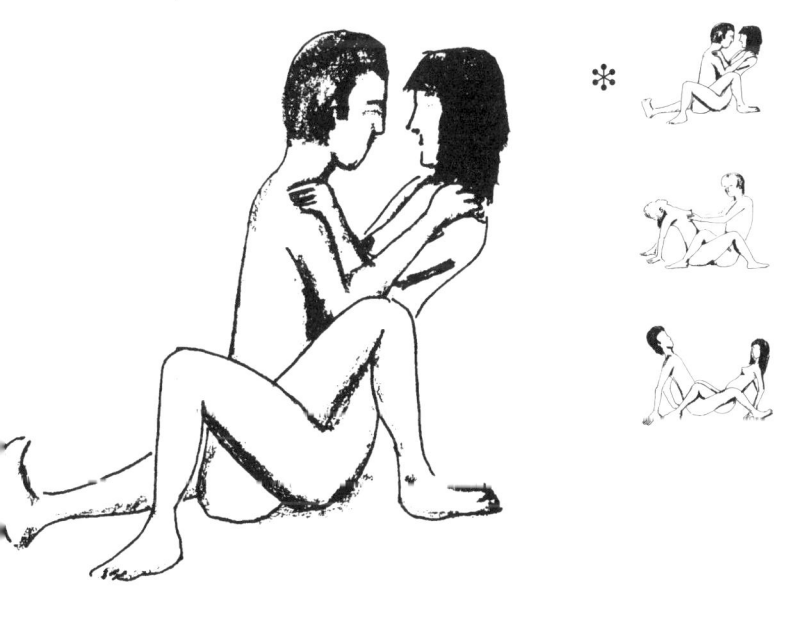

Sextrology

6-2 When one of the couple remains upright and the other leans his/her back backward (supported by his/her arms or by the other one's arms) to form a 45-degree angle.

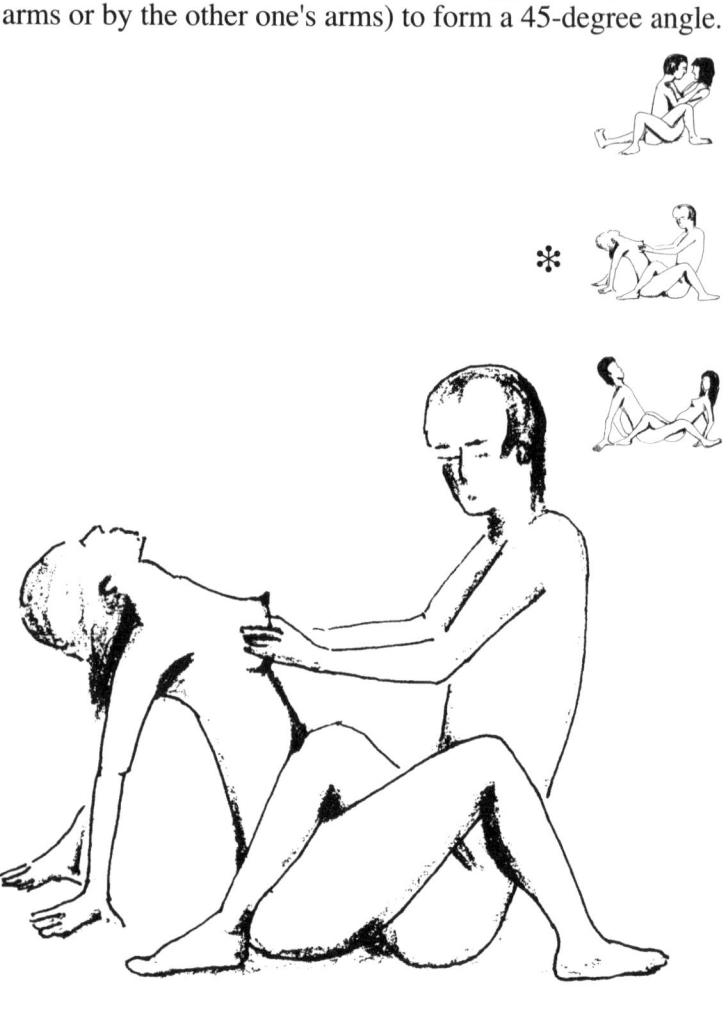

36

Sextrology

6-3 When both partners lean backward (supported by holding each other or by leaning on their arms) to form an angle that is close to 90 degrees (like the letter V).

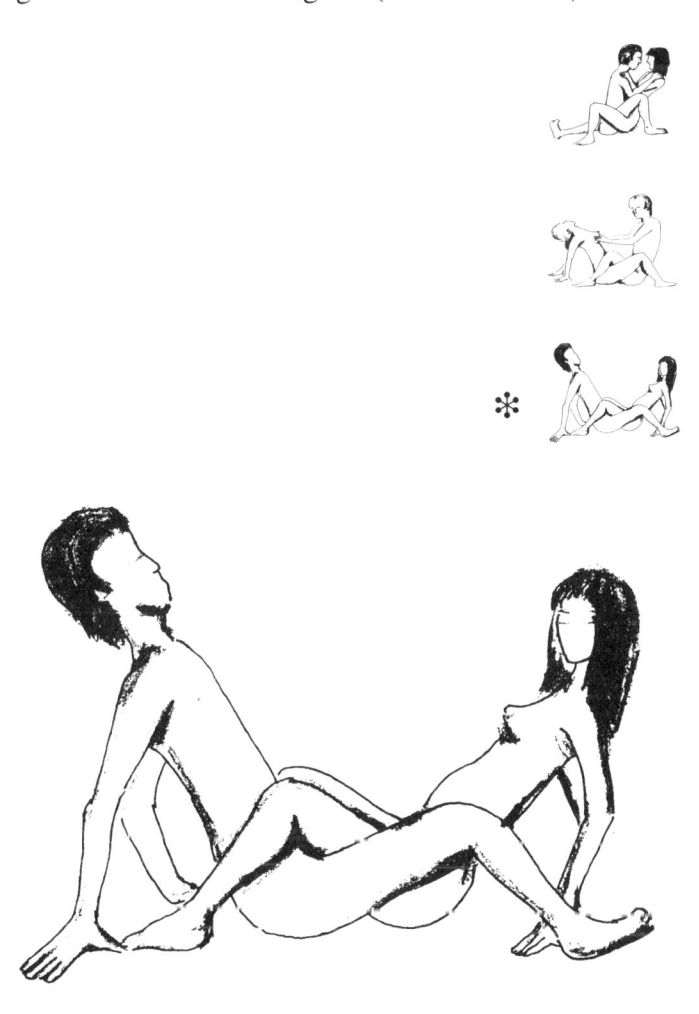

Sextrology

7. In the seventh basic position, both partners are in a sitting position, the man serving as a "chair" and the woman sitting on him, with her face or the side of her body turned toward him. As in the sixth position, a lot of contact between their mouths is possible as well as extensive use of their hands. In this position, their legs are on top of each other, and the position of the legs determines the different variations. In the East, these positions are performed with the help of large pillows. In the West, they can be performed on a chair or armchair.

7-1 When the man sits supported by his arms or holding the woman's body, and the woman sits facing him, her thighs above his thighs, her legs open at the sides of his body, and her face turned toward him.

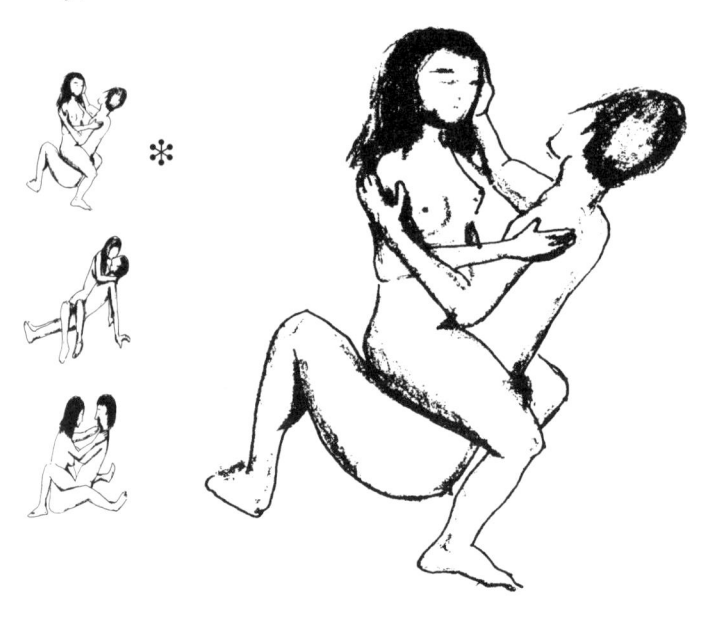

Sextrology

7-2 When the man sits supported by his arms or holding the woman's body, and the woman sits with her side facing him, her thighs above his thighs, both her legs turned to one side and close together.

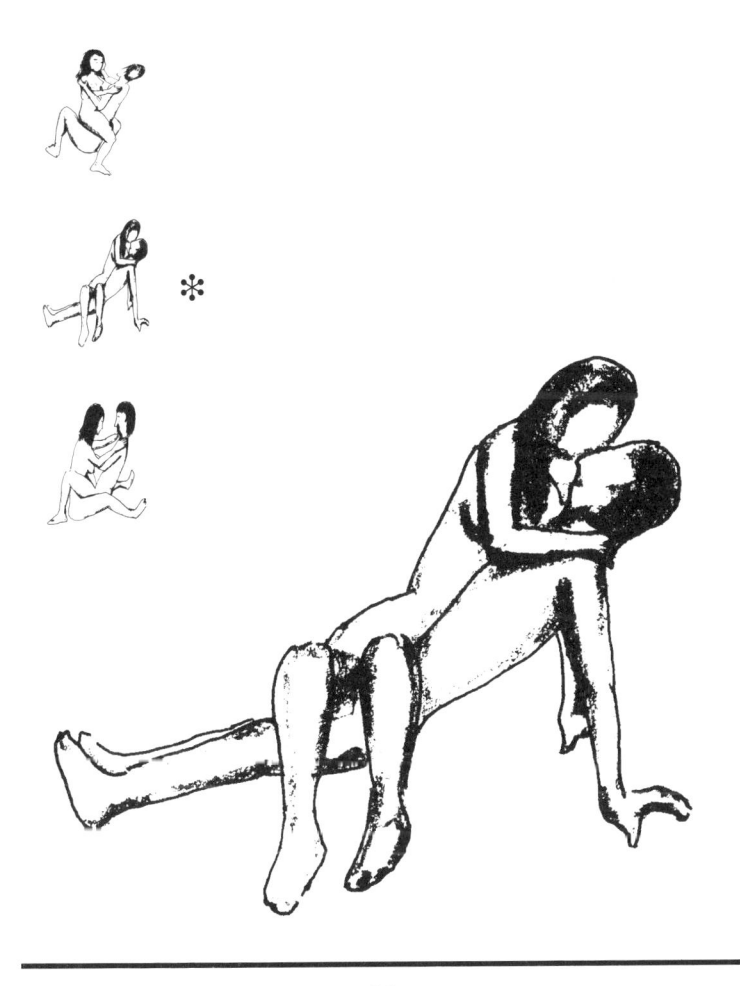

Sextrology

7-3 When the man sits supported by his arms or holding the woman's body, and the woman sits facing him, one of her thighs below one of his, and her other leg above his other thigh. (Pliancy is required in order to perform this position properly.)

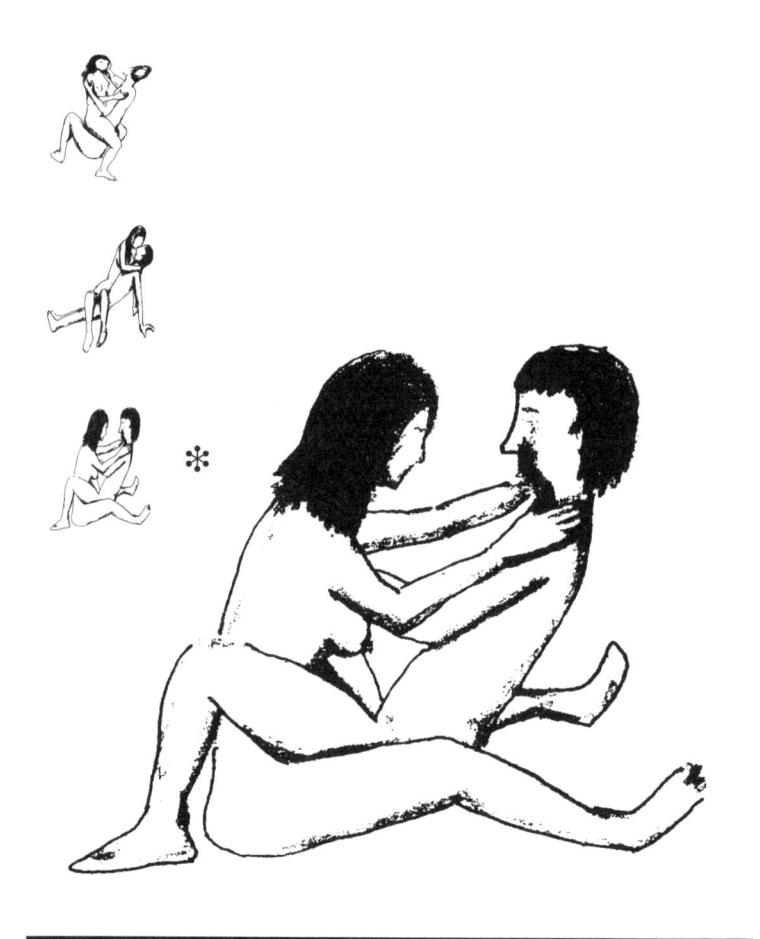

40

Sextrology

8. In the eighth basic position, both partners sit, except that this time the woman's back is turned toward the man (like spoons fitting into each other). In this position, when the man has support for his back, he has the opportunity to use his hands and mouth enthusiastically. The man sits with spread legs, and the woman sits between his legs and close to him. Alternatively, he wraps his legs around the woman's body. The variations on this position are determined by the angles of the woman's body, while the man hardly changes his position:

8-1 When both partners are close together (the woman's back against the man's chest), to form a 90-degree angle with the mattress.

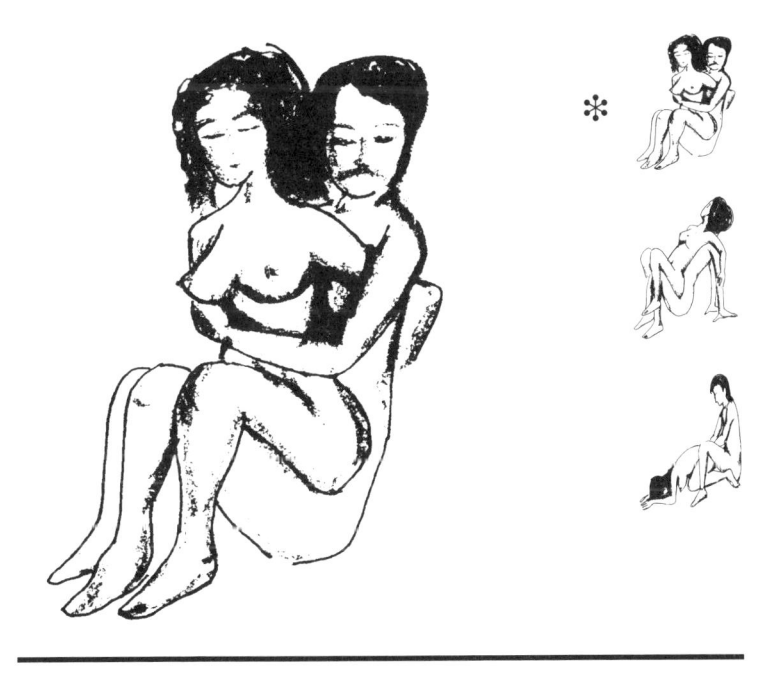

Sextrology

8-2 When the woman bends backward slightly (the man naturally leans back slightly, too), her body is close to the man's body.

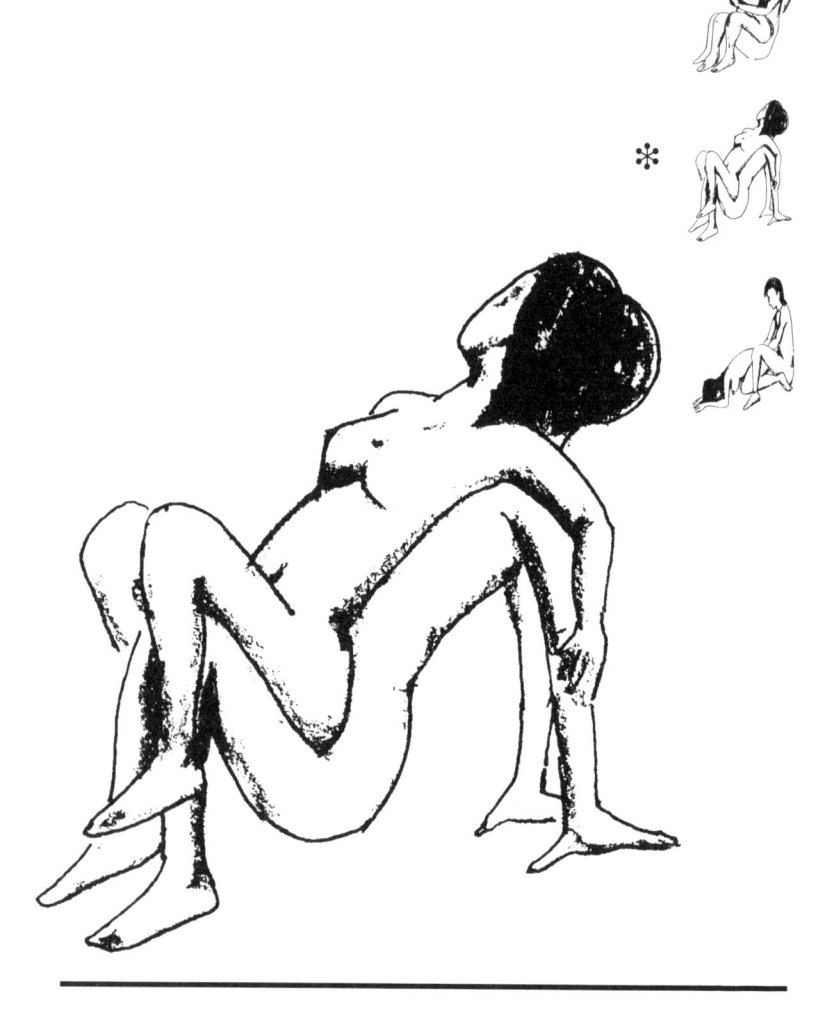

Sextrology

8-3 When the woman leans forward until only her bottom touches the man's body (an angle of almost 90 degrees).

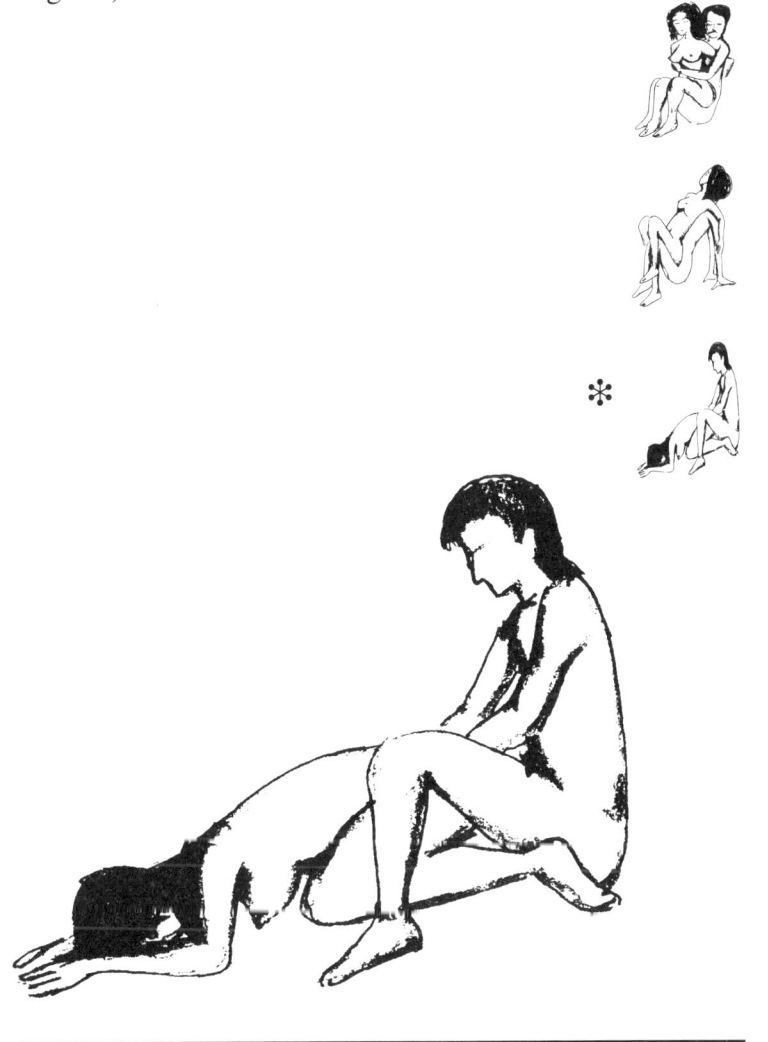

Sextrology

9. The ninth basic position is the most ancient position to appear in the dawn of civilization. This position, as you will see, ensures that the man is able to see what is going on around him the whole time and be alert to danger. In the West, the position is nicknamed "doggy style," while in the East it is generally called "the Tao position." In this position, the man controls the pace of the sexual act. In the various cultures of the East, there are associations between this position and homosexual love. The woman can place herself in different positions, but it is the position of the man that determines the variations:

9-1 When the man sits on his knees and ankles, his bottom resting on his ankles and his arms pulling the woman toward him.

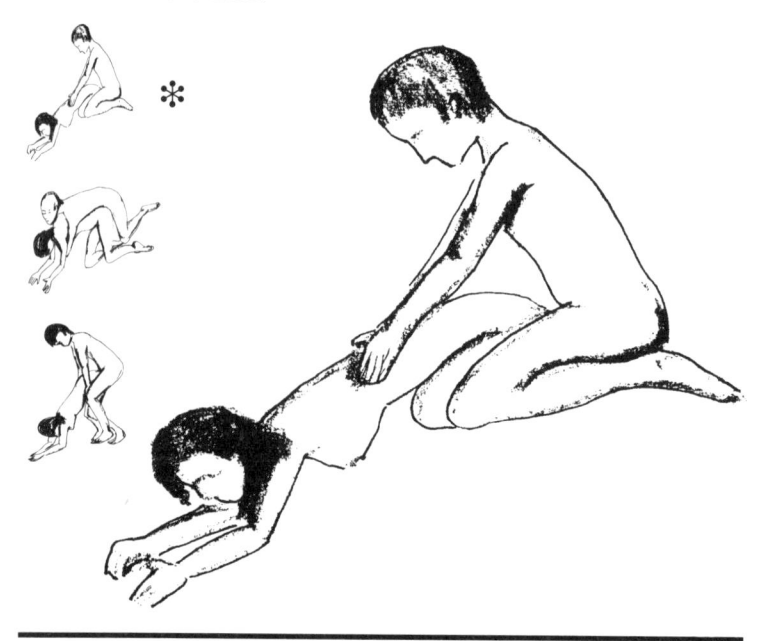

Sextrology

9-2 When the man is on his knees, holding the woman, his stomach leaning against her bottom.

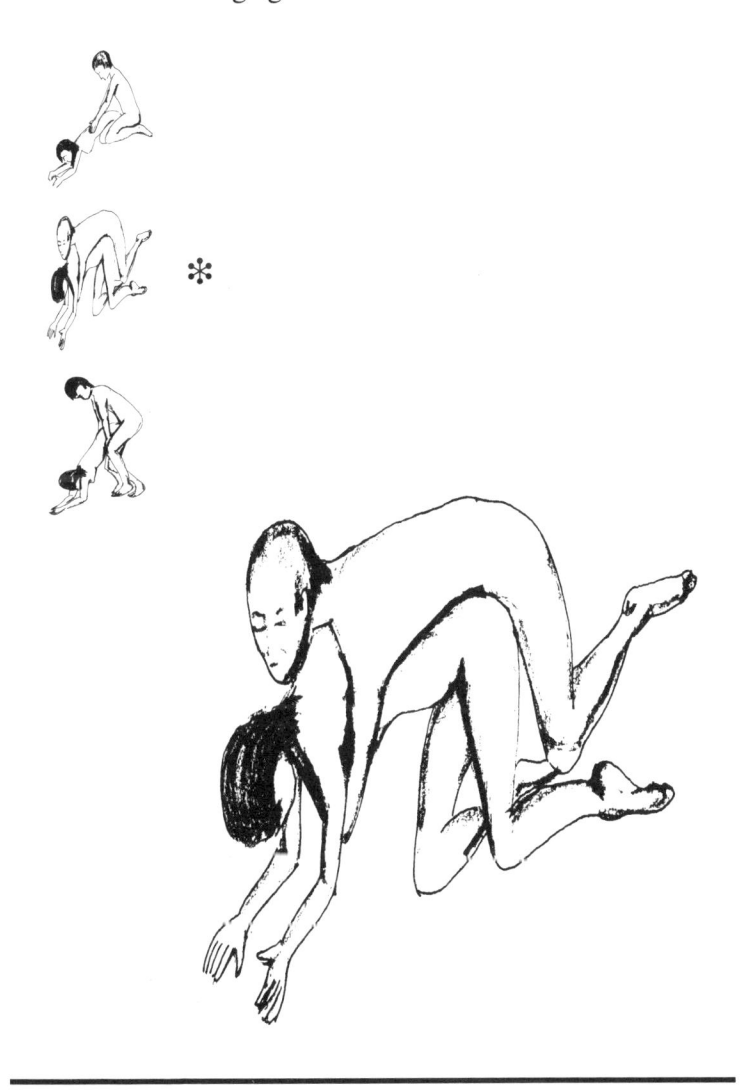

Sextrology

9-3 When the man is standing up (with straight or bent legs) and leaning with his arms on the woman from "above."

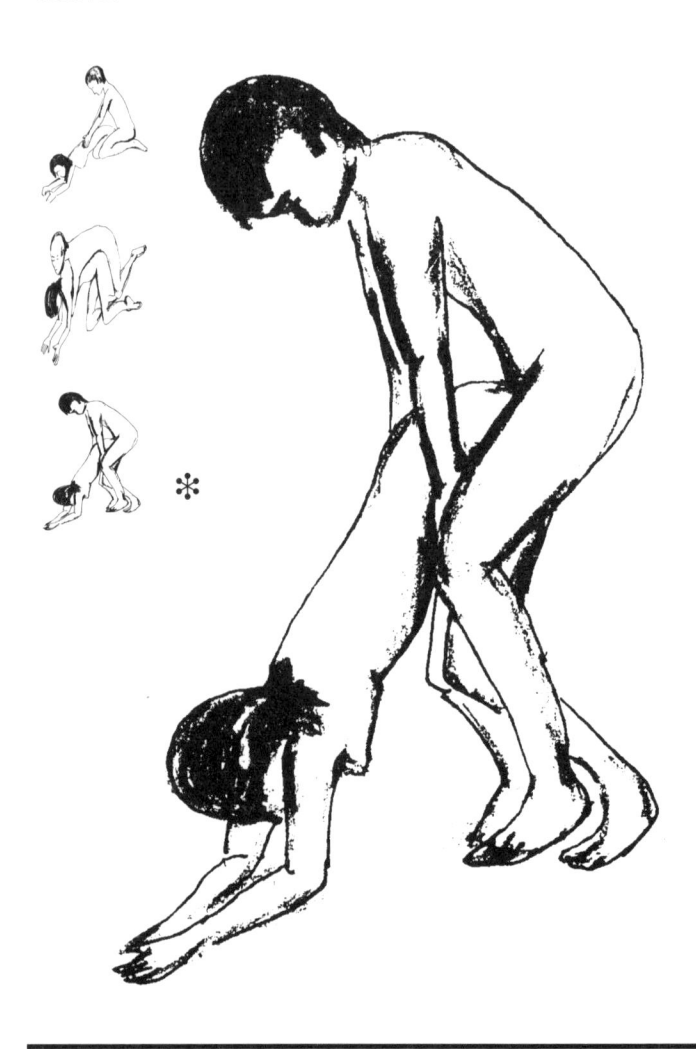

Sextrology

10. The tenth basic position is the first of the standing positions. Standing positions require physical fitness and good compatibility between the partners from the point of view of both physique and sexual experience. These positions afford the partners a great deal of intense sexual pleasure - so long as they learn to know the rhythms, movements, and body angles that are special to these positions. In the tenth basic position, the man stands with his body upright (he can lean against a wall) with the woman on his body without touching the floor or the wall, her arms clasped tightly around his neck or on his shoulders. The position of the woman's legs and the placement of the man's hands while he is supporting her body determine the variations on this basic position:

10-1 When the man's arms are at his sides, supporting the woman's legs, which are bent and spread (it is she who is actually moving her pelvis, as if sitting on a saddle).

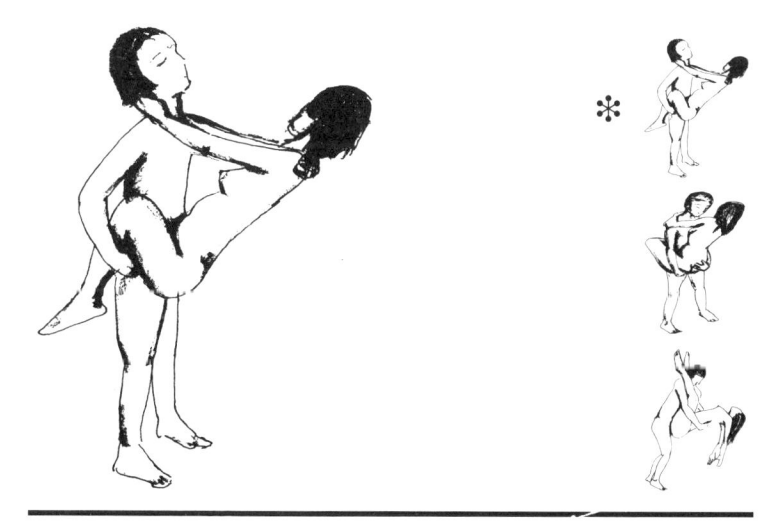

Sextrology

10-2 When the woman's legs, spread, are wrapped around the man's waist, and the man clasps her bottom from below and presses her body to his.

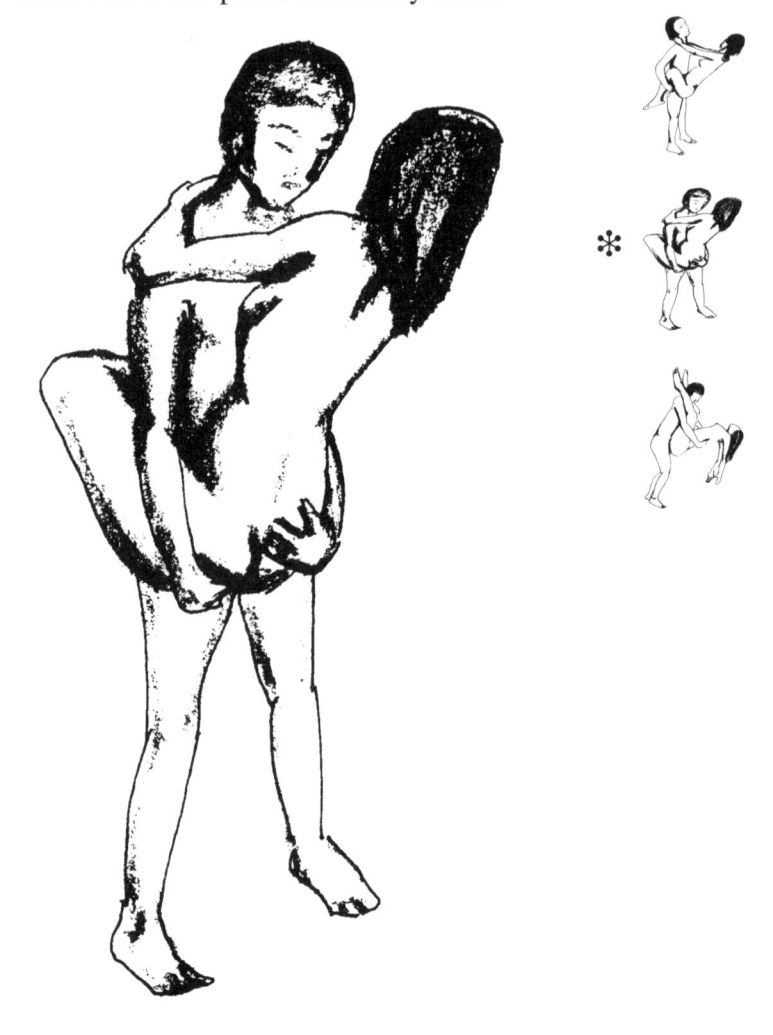

Sextrology

10-3 When the woman's legs are placed (straight or bent) on the man's shoulders (a lot of pliancy is required for this) and the man's arms are around her waist, pulling the woman to him (the position of the legs makes the union of the genitals difficult, and the man must pull the woman to him). When there is compatibility between the man and the woman, and the woman can maintain this position with her legs bent, she can move her body and set the pace.

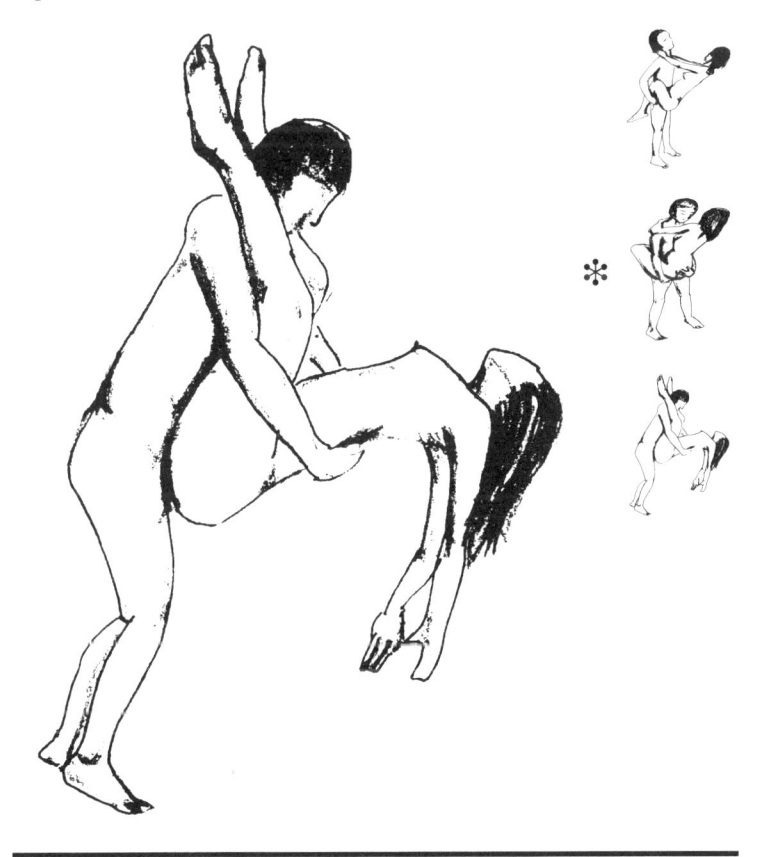

Sextrology

11. The following basic position is also a standing position, except that this time the man's legs can be either straight or bent and he leans against a (real or imaginary) high chair, table edge, or pillar. The woman sits on him (as in the seventh basic position). His bent thighs support the woman's body, and she is not suspended as in the previous position. Her arms can support themselves on his neck, shoulders, back or hips. The position of the woman's body determines the variations:

11-1 When the woman faces the man, and both of her legs are spread and bent at his sides.

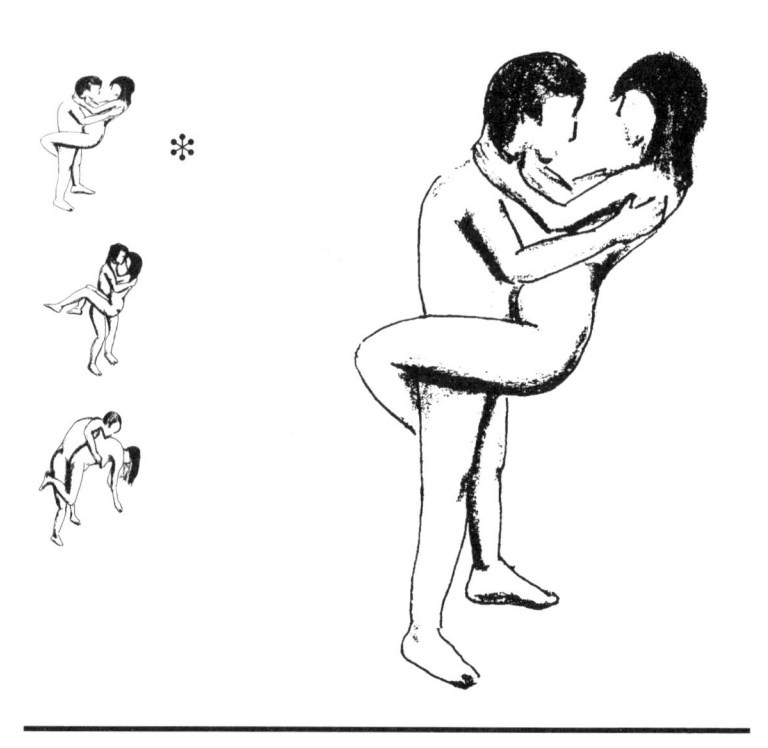

Sextrology

11-2 When the woman faces sideways, her legs bent and turned to one side of the man's body (it is not easy to achieve sexual union in this position).

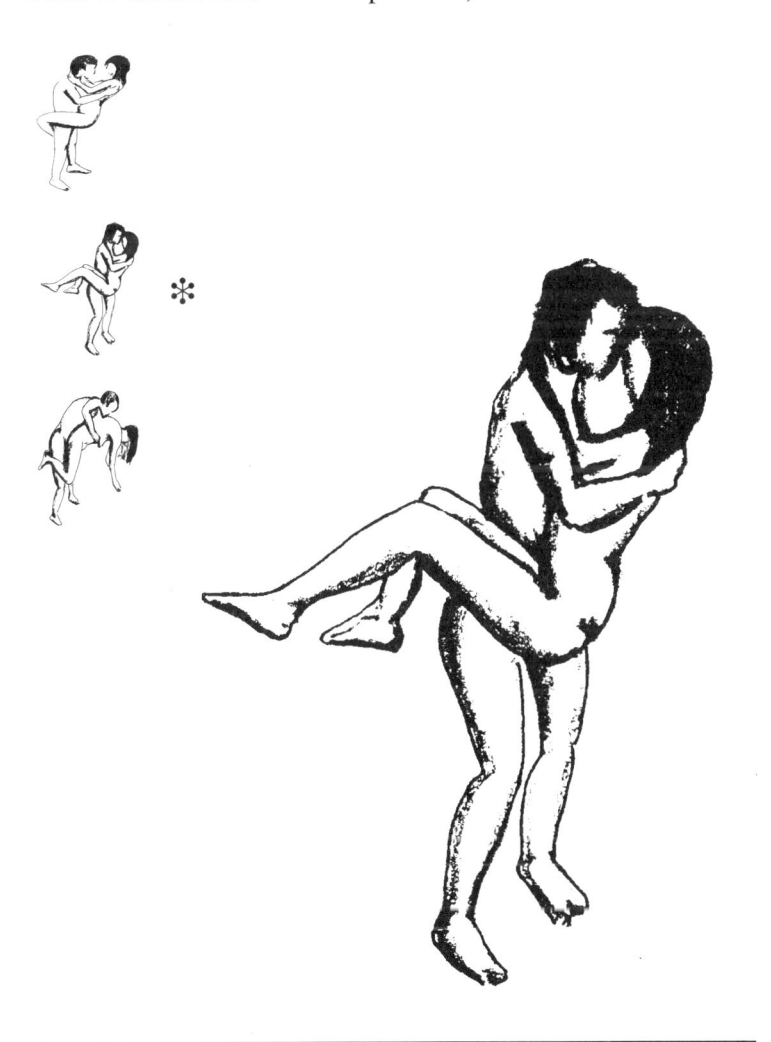

Sextrology

11-3 When the woman's back faces the man and he holds her tightly, and her legs are bent at the sides of the man's body.

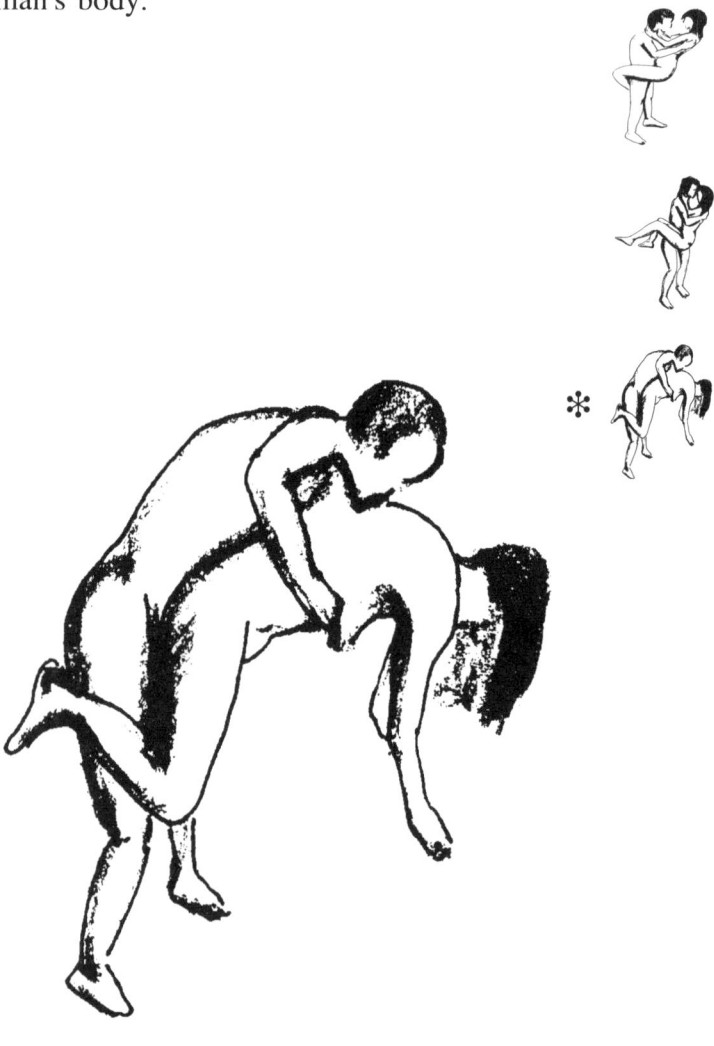

Sextrology

12. The last basic position is also a standing position, except that this time a lot of pliancy is required, as is compatibility and trust between the partners. In this basic position, the man stands (without support) and serves as a "trunk" on which the woman climbs. He holds her thighs or hips - she has no solid basis and does not hold onto his body. This position is characterized by the fact that the woman's head is ultimately lower than her pelvis, as well as by the fact that in this basic position the woman performs a transition after union has been achieved in order to get into the "final" stage of the position. The variations here are:

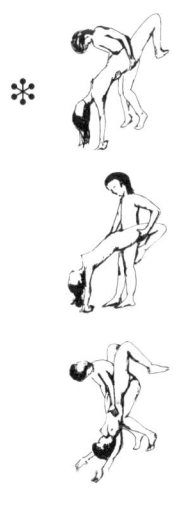

Sextrology

12-1 When the man and the woman are face to face. The man holds the woman's bottom and helps her climb up him while she clasps his neck. After union, the woman bends her body backward, releases her grip, and lowers her body to the floor until her arms are supported on the floor, while the man holds onto her The woman's legs are as straight as she can make them, and she tries to hold them in a straight line with her body (she generally has to bend her knees a bit). Pliancy is required to perform this position, and the man must be careful while the woman bends her body backward and "falls" to the ground. The accepted Eastern approach describes the position as a stage of "climbing" followed by a stage of "falling," but it is possible to achieve this position from the "final stage" as well - that is, the woman lies on her back, and the man lifts her legs into the final position and penetrates her - without spoiling the pleasure.

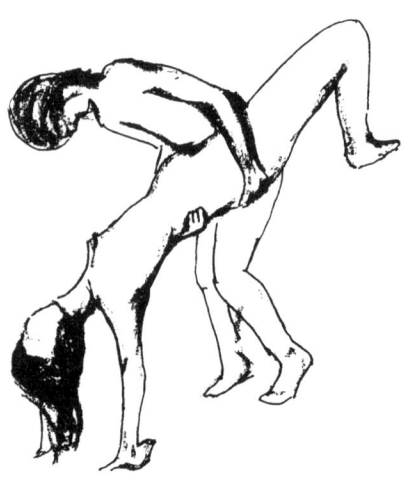

Sextrology

12-2 When the man stands firm, and the woman climbs up him (as in position 11-3), and while she is doing so the man grasps her waist and bends her body toward the ground until her arms are leaning on the floor. The man holds her legs and fits his body into hers. The woman bends her legs so that her feet press onto the man's thighs or buttocks. Here, too, the final stage can be reached without bending the woman to the ground, from the basic position of 9-3, for instance.

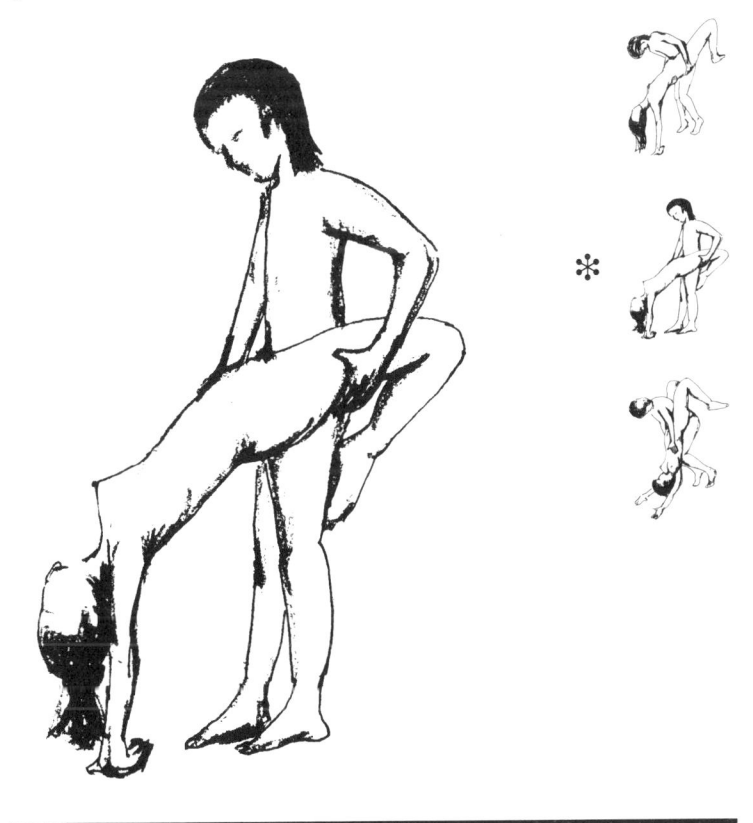

Sextrology

12-3 When the woman's shoulders are on the mattress, and her back and legs point straight up, as if she is doing a shoulder stand. The man stands on his feet, legs spread, and holds her legs in his arms, while he places his body between her spread legs. From here, he lowers himself toward the woman until union is achieved. Although the description of this position seems complicated, it is very simple to do. It can be achieved, of course, from position 12-1 too (that is, by bending the body down and half a twist), but that requires great pliancy. There are many variations on this position, but the main point is for the woman to create a strong, broad basis on the floor with her shoulders.

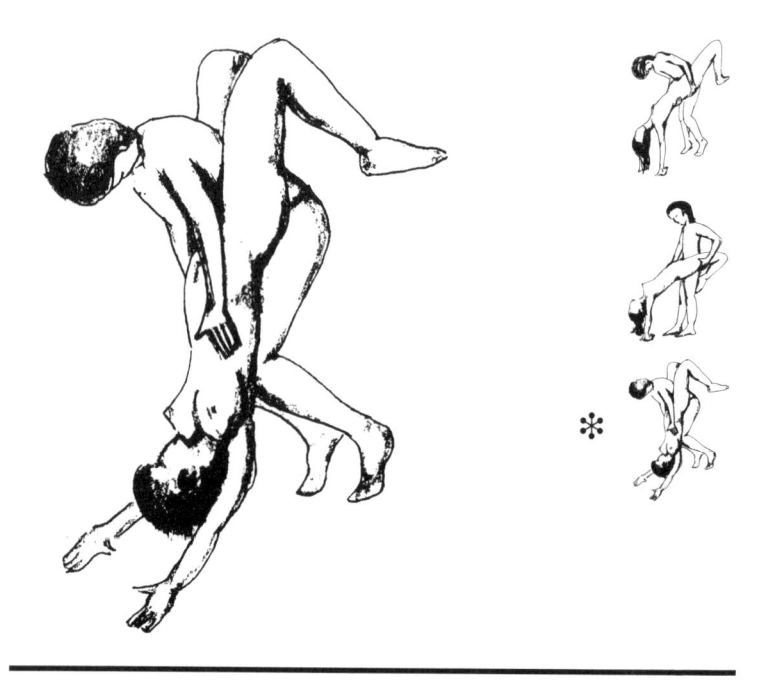

A. Table showing preference for positions according to signs of the Zodiac

	Man	Woman
Aries	2-1 9-2 3-3 8-2	9-1 3-1 5-2 2-2
Taurus	8-1 4-3 9-3 7-1	1-3 11-2 10-1 6-2
Gemini	5-1 1-2 6-3 9-1	12-1 7-2 11-1 8-1
Cancer	1-3 5-3 2-3 11-3	9-2 2-3 12-2 5-3
Leo	8-2 9-3 2-1 6-1	10-2 5-1 6-3 7-3
Virgo	8-3 7-1 6-2 3-1	8-1 1-1 10-3 6-2
Libra	7-2 8-1 10-2 3-2	10-2 11-3 12-2 6-1
Scorpio	4-2 1-2 11-2 12-2	7-3 9-3 5-2 8-2
Sagittarius	5-1 1-1 4-1 11-1	2-1 3-2 9-1 4-2
Capricorn	12-1 10-1 2-2 10-3	1-3 2-1 4-3 3-3
Aquarius	3-2 12-3 7-3 9-2	1-1 4-1 12-3 7-1
Pisces	5-2 8-3 6-3 10-2	4-3 1-2 8-3 3-2

This table shows the four positions favored by each sign (men and women separately). The order of the positions in each sign is of no importance (that is, each of the four positions is equally favored).

B. Table showing which signs favor which positions

	Men	**Women**
1-1	Sagittarius	Virgo Aquarius
1-2	Gemini Scorpio	Pisces
1-3	Cancer	Taurus Capricorn
2-1	Aries Leo	Sagittarius Capricorn
2-2	Capricorn	Aries
2-3	Cancer	Cancer
3-1	Virgo	Aries
3-2	Aquarius Libra	Sagittarius Pisces
3-3	Aries	Capricorn
4-1	Sagittarius	Aquarius
4-2	Scorpio	Sagittarius
4-3	Taurus	Capricorn Pisces
5-1	Gemini Sagittarius	Leo
5-2	Pisces	Aries Scorpio
5-3	Cancer	Cancer
6-1	Leo	Libra
6-2	Virgo	Taurus Virgo
6-3	Gemini Pisces	Leo

Sextrology

7-1	Taurus Virgo	Aquarius
7-2	Libra	Gemini
7-3	Aquarius	Leo Scorpio
8-1	Taurus Libra	Gemini Virgo
8-2	Aries Leo	Scorpio
8-3	Virgo Pisces	Pisces
9-1	Gemini	Aries Sagittarius
9-2	Aries Aquarius	Cancer
9-3	Taurus Leo	Scorpio
10-1	Capricorn	Taurus
10-2	Pisces Libra	Leo Libra
10-3	Capricorn	Virgo
11-1	Sagittarius	Gemini
11-2	Scorpio	Taurus
11-3	Cancer	Libra
12-1	Capricorn	Gemini
12-2	Scorpio	Cancer Libra
12-3	Aquarius	Aquarius

This table shows which signs favor which of the 36 positions.

Sextrology

C. Table showing the perfect sexual compatibilities for men

Men	with Women
Aries	Sagittarius, Capricorn, Scorpio, Cancer
Taurus	Capricorn, Pisces, Aquarius, Gemini, Virgo, Scorpio
Gemini	Pisces, Leo, Aries, Sagittarius
Cancer	Taurus, Capricorn, Cancer, Libra
Leo	Sagittarius, Capricorn, Libra, Scorpio
Virgo	Aries, Taurus, Virgo, Aquarius, Pisces
Libra	Sagittarius, Pisces, Gemini, Virgo, Leo, Libra
Scorpio	Pisces, Sagittarius, Taurus, Cancer, Libra
Sagittarius	Virgo, Aquarius, Leo, Gemini
Capricorn	Aries, Taurus, Virgo, Gemini
Aquarius	Sagittarius, Pisces, Leo, Scorpio, Cancer, Aquarius
Pisces	Aries, Scorpio, Pisces, Leo, Libra

D. Table showing the perfect sexual compatibilities for women

Women	with Men
Aries	Capricorn, Virgo, Pisces, Gemini
Taurus	Cancer, Virgo, Capricorn, Scorpio
Gemini	Libra, Taurus, Sagittarius, Capricorn
Cancer	Cancer, Aries, Aquarius, Scorpio
Leo	Gemini, Sagittarius, Pisces, Aquarius, Libra
Virgo	Sagittarius, Taurus, Libra, Capricorn
Libra	Leo, Pisces, Libra, Cancer, Scorpio
Scorpio	Pisces, Aquarius, Aries, Leo, Taurus
Sagittarius	Aries, Leo, Aquarius, Libra, Scorpio, Gemini
Capricorn	Cancer, Aries, Leo, Taurus
Aquarius	Sagittarius, Taurus, Virgo, Aquarius
Pisces	Gemini, Scorpio, Aquarius, Libra, Taurus, Virgo, Pisces

Matching Lingam and Yoni

The basic division of men and women in the East, according to the Indian books, the *Kama Sutra* and the *Ananga Ranga*, is according to the size of the lingam, the male sex organ, or the depth of the yoni, the female sex organ.

In men, the dimensions are:
Rabbit size - 3 inches or about 8 centimeters in length
Ox size - 4-5 inches or about 11-13 centimeters in length.
Horse size - 6-7 inches or about 15-18 centimeters in length.

In women, the dimensions are:
Deer size - 3 inches or about 8 centimeters in depth.
Mare size - 4-5 inches or about 11-13 centimeters in depth.
Elephant size - 6-7 inches or about 15-18 centimeters in depth.

Different sources give different dimensions, and sometimes the names differ. However, this is the most widely accepted division. The measurements refer to organs in a state of sexual arousal.

Sextrology

The greatest compatibility occurs when the sizes match: rabbit with deer, ox with mare, and horse with elephant.

Near compatibility occurs when there is no substantial discrepancy between the dimensions of the man and the woman. In other words, rabbit with mare, ox with deer, ox with elephant, horse with mare.

A lack of compatibility occurs when the discrepancy is the greatest between the man and the woman: rabbit with elephant or horse with deer.

(It is therefore obvious that the ox and the mare are in the best situation, and in the East, they are described as "the rivers of passion," that is, they adapt themselves to the channel in which they flow, like a river.)

The aim of this book is to ensure a perfect union between the members of a couple whose dimensions do not match, taking into account the sexual temperament of each one.

In the questionnaire that each person, male or female, in each sign is asked to complete, the male reader is asked to define himself as a rabbit, ox, or horse, while the female reader is asked to define herself as a deer, mare, or elephant.

After adding up the questionnaire scores, every reader is ranked in one of three possibilities, and receives a numerical grade. This grade enables the reader to attain the perfect match between man and woman.

In this way, every reader can find, in addition to

compatibility between the signs, compatibility according to the sexual temperament or nature.

The basic principle is simple - the smaller the difference, the greater the compatibility. We will see that this compatibility of sexual temperament can occasionally overcome a lack of compatibility in size.

For instance, a rabbit with an elephant is not a recommended union, but different situations must be examined: in the case of a "weak" rabbit with the number 1 and a "strong" elephant with a number 9, the difference is 8 and is extremely blatant. In contrast, a "strong" rabbit with a number 7 will feel comfortable with an "average" elephant with a number 6, and the difference between him and a "strong" elephant with a number 9 or a "weak" elephant with a number 3 is also not so blatant. The difference between a number 7 rabbit and a number 9 elephant is smaller than between a number 3 horse and a number 6 elephant, for example.

The best compatibilities are the identical ones: 1/1, 2/2, and so on, up to 9/9.

Reasonable compatibilities are the ones where the difference between them is no greater than 3, that is: 1/2, 1/3, 1/4, 5/6, 8/9, 7/9, and so on.

Problematic compatibilities are the ones where the difference between them is between 4 and 6, that is: 1/5, 7/3, 5/9, 2/8 and so on.

Difficult compatibilities are the ones where the difference between them is 7 or 8, that is: 1/8, 1/9, 2/9.

According to Western Astrology

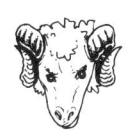

Aries

The Aries person likes to be on his own - after all, he is the first sign of the Zodiac - and he is not in a hurry to establish a relationship with a member of the opposite sex, or to get married.

Aries people are inclined to play around, to indulge in non-committal sex, and to masturbate extensively. In spite of this, they are considered to be attractive lovers, especially after they have gone through adulthood.

The Aries person has a charming personality, and when he indulges in sex - either with himself or with a partner - he does so with all his heart. He is a persistent but charming suitor, and after deciding that he wishes to establish a relationship with a particular partner, he won't leave that person alone until his wish is granted.

The Aries male's crisis point occurs in two cases. Sometimes he will hesitate to engage in sexual intercourse with his partner, even though all the appropriate circumstances prevail. Moreover, he is capable of fleeing from the threat of marriage - even to the point of deserting his bride at the altar!

After he gets married, the Aries male spends a lot of time away from home (although he is not necessarily cheating on his wife). He is quite a good lover, and tries to satisfy his wife. However, the sexual relations between them will be frozen at the level they reached before their

According to Western Astrology

marriage. The lack of development in their sexual relations is liable to lead to sexual boredom and crises in the couple's lives.

The Aries female is direct in her approach to sex, courting, and marriage. She tries to be pleasant to men, and does not have many inhibitions about sex.

The Aries female will be among the first of her contemporaries to lose her virginity, and among the first to marry. However, in the generally brief period of time between the loss of her virginity and her marriage, she will be with a lot of men and enjoy a variety of sexual relations.

The Aries male

The Aries male is ruled by the star of war. The man is average in height, with strong organs and superb physical fitness. The Aries male's penis is average in size, but he knows how to use it skillfully as a real weapon.

The Aries male considers the conquest of his partner to be his primary objective, so he rushes to push his sword into her scabbard. This is not a cease-fire, however - but rather the beginning of a pleasurable and enjoyable battle.

The Aries male sees sexual intercourse itself as his main aim, and all the sexual foreplay - from hugging and kissing onward - are just means to the end.

The Aries male is quick to fire, but, lucky for him, also quick to recover and cock his weapon once more.

Important: An Aries male whose sexual performance fails because of erection failure will lose his confidence for a long time.

According to sextrology, the favorite positions of the Aries male are 2-1, 9-2, 3-3, 8-2 (not necessarily in that order). For details, see the chapter on positions.

The Aries female

The Aries female is well aware of her external appearance, and flaunts her femininity continually. She uses her beauty and her body to reach the man of her heart... and then she surrenders unconditionally to his weapon!

She always adapts to her lover's rhythm, and in actual intercourse forgets herself and exposes the real Aries in her - unbridled passion.

She likes well-endowed men who are well versed in all the arts of the bedroom. Quality is more important to her than quantity in anything pertaining to sexual intercourse, even though she prefers body to spirit in the man himself.

In her prime, the Aries female adapts herself body and mind to the man who both loves her and is her lover. She will not break up with him easily, and will resort to anything to keep him. During intercourse, her ability to adapt to any sexual rhythm the man may set turns her into the playmate of choice...

In contrast, her tendency to make comparisons between her lovers may alienate men.

The Aries female is orgasmic by nature, and with the right partner, will reach stunning multiple orgasms easily. Her pubic region is her pleasure center.

Sextrology

Important: *The Aries female can reach heights of pleasure in intercourse with many men... but for love, she must find the one and only man for her!*

According to sextrology, the favorite positions of the Aries female are 9-1, 3-1, 5-2, 2-2 (not necessarily in that order).
For details, see the chapter on positions.

According to Western Astrology

The relationship between the *Aries* male/female and the members of the other signs:

Aries:
A brief affair, focusing mainly on a quick roll in the hay, quick satisfaction.

Taurus:
Bad sex because of too many physical and mental differences.

Gemini:
Mutual fruitfulness - the man turns the woman on, and the woman turns the man on.

Cancer:
Contradictory aims - one side wants bed, the other side wants marriage.

Leo:
A life full of passion, both in and out of bed.

Virgo:
A life of master and slave - and its sexual derivatives, of course.

Libra:
Mutual respect, sometimes to the detriment of performance in bed.

According to Western Astrology

Scorpio:
Friction that interrupts regular sexual activity.

Sagittarius:
A happy life, expressed in sex, too.

Capricorn:
Too many differences.

Aquarius:
Intellectual interest distracts the mind from any real activity...

Pisces:
Stormy rows lead to unforgettable moments of reconciliation.

Sextrology

The aim of this questionnaire is to determine how well the **Aries man** matches the sextrological profile presented in this book.

Answer only Yes or No for each question. It is mandatory to answer all the questions.

Yes/No   1. Do you define yourself as active and dynamic in a relationship that includes sex?

Yes/No   2. Are you prepared to take risks in the field of sex?

Yes/No   3. Do you consider sex as a sports contest in which there is a winner and a loser?

Yes/No   4. Do you prefer immediate gratification - that is, have sex quickly - or do you prefer to delay gratification - that is, build a relationship slowly?

Yes/No   5. While having sex, do you think more about your own satisfaction than about your partner's satisfaction?

Yes/No   6. Do you define yourself as having a fierce desire for sex?

Yes/No   7. Do you prefer to be the first (that is, the first man in a woman's life) to being another in a row of men who have already "ploughed the field"?

Add up the positive answers.

If you answered "Yes" to one or two of the questions, you match the profile of the Aries man "poorly."

If you answered "Yes" to three, four, or five of the questions, you match the profile of the Aries man "in an average and normal way."

Sextrology

If you answered "Yes" to six or seven of the questions, you match the profile of the Aries man "well."

Now we will add the questionnaire that the expert in Indian astrology and in the *Kama Sutra* would have constructed:

Do you define yourself as a rabbit, an ox, or a horse?

Now find the category to which you belong by following the simple procedure below:
(1) Circle the category (Rabbit, Ox, or Horse) that describes you.
(2) Circle the category (Poorly, Average & normal, or Well) according to your questionnaire score.
(3) Find the number where the two above categories meet. This number is your sextrological matching number.

	Rabbit	**Ox**	**Horse**
Poorly	1	2	3
Average & normal	4	5	6
Well	7	8	9

Sextrology

The aim of this questionnaire is to determine how well the **Aries woman** matches the sextrological profile presented in this book.

Answer only Yes or No for each question. It is mandatory to answer all the questions.

Yes/No 1. Do you believe that the next man in your life will be better sexually than the previous one (or the present one)?

Yes/No 2. Do you believe that sex would be more pleasurable with a man who is younger than you?

Yes/No 3. Are you prepared to try - at least theoretically - anything in the field of sex?

Yes/No 4. Is it important for you to be the one and only woman in the heart of the man you love?

Yes/No 5. Do you think that sex declines over time as a matter of course?

Yes/No 6. Would you always prefer a man who is experienced in sex to one who is inexperienced?

Yes/No 7. Do you believe that in comparison to your girlfriends you are "much better in bed" than they are?

Add up the positive answers.

If you answered "Yes" to one or two of the questions, you match the profile of the Aries woman "poorly."

If you answered "Yes" to three, four, or five of the questions, you match the profile of the Aries woman "in an average and normal way."

If you answered "Yes" to six or seven of the questions, you match the profile of the Aries woman "well."

Sextrology

Now we will add the questionnaire that the expert in Indian astrology and in the *Kama Sutra* would have constructed:

Do you define yourself as a deer, a mare, or an elephant?

Now find the category to which you belong by following the simple procedure below:

(1) Circle the category (Deer, Mare, or Elephant) that describes you.

(2) Circle the category (Poorly, Average & normal, or Well) according to you questionnaire score.

(3) Find the number where the two above categories meet. This number is your sextrological matching number.

	Deer	**Mare**	**Elephant**
Poorly	1	2	3
Average & normal	4	5	6
Well	7	8	9

According to Western Astrology

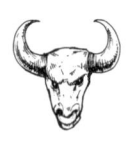

Taurus

The Taurus male is very considered in all his ways and conduct, and this applies to his approach to sex, love, and marriage as well. He is not tempted by every opportunity that falls into his lap.

He chooses his partners meticulously, out of considerations that are not just sexual or emotional. For instance, a Taurus male is capable of masturbating before a date with a girl - not for his pleasure, but in order to remain in control of himself in her presence. He is a clumsy but thorough lover.

A Taurus male who has set his sights on a partner finds it hard to take no for an answer. After he has convinced himself that he wants the girl, he will consider any refusal to be hurtful, and is even capable of becoming violent.

A Taurus male who proposes to a girl and is turned down virtually sees a red flag being waved in front of him!

When he wants to get married, the Taurus male chooses a girl who suits his status, and is faithful to her all his life.

Generally speaking, he loses his virginity the easy way - in a brothel or with girls who "put out." His active imagination is limited, and he draws his knowledge from books or magazines, in most cases.

The Taurus female directs her way in love, pursuit, and sex toward one objective - to marry the right guy, and as quickly as possible. She guards herself against a reputation of "putting out" or "sleeping around", but considers sex to be an acceptable means of accomplishing her objectives.

After she has achieved her aim, the Taurus female will be faithful to her husband, even though she is possessive and jealous in everything to do with other women.

When one member of a married couple is a Taurus person, they have a stable marriage that lasts for a long time, in spite of minor disputes and arguments.

The Taurus male

The Taurus male is ruled by the star of pleasure, and he is equipped with everything necessary to achieve his pleasures. His body is strong, his muscles are hard, his physical fitness is excellent, and he has a long, solid penis, with a long range of activity.

He sees sexual intercourse as a pleasure in itself, and enjoys foreplay as much as the act itself. He takes his time during intercourse and pleasures his partner. By nature, the Taurus male comes once, and after that he will bow out of the game.

In spite of his talents, the Taurus man is not crazy about sexual activity, and sometimes prefers more moderate pleasures to sex.

***Important:** The Taurus male is unimaginative by nature, and in order to reach real climaxes, his partner has to make an effort to use her imagination.*

According to sextrology, the favorite positions of the Taurus male are 8-1, 4-3, 9-3, 7-1 (not necessarily in that order).
For details, see the chapter on positions.

The Taurus female

The man who chanced to get hold of a Taurus female will remember her forever - positively or negatively! The Taurus female is always ready for sex, and will make the most of any opportunity to vary her sex life...

But she is also the one who quickly tires of monotonous, repetitive activity - even if her partner is a highly potent guy... but devoid of imagination!

The Taurus female, who is not particularly orgasmic, learns to bring her body to a climax by becoming acquainted with its rhythm and her erogenous zones. That's why she needs so much variety in her sex life.

As a rule, the Taurus female prefers variety with one lover blessed with a fertile imagination... but in no case will she give up on her right to pleasure in bed. If the guy who is with her does not try hard enough, she will not hesitate to seek variety in other beds.

The Taurus female is in the habit of clasping the man in her arms and legs during intercourse. For this reason, she does not expose her posterior to his tool very often. She is proud of her breasts and uses them constantly in the game of love. In contrast, she is afraid that her posterior may repel the guy.

The suitable partner, the highly imaginative man, will gain a great deal of support from the Taurus female - not only in her willingness to adopt every variation of position and rhythm, but also by cheering on his penis vigorously, if need be, until it is erect.

The Taurus female is extremely circumspect in "publicizing" her acts of intercourse, and in order to get hold of a good lover, she is prepared to ignore "marginal" problems such as the guy's wife, age, or status.

Important: *The Taurus female is "submissive" toward the man who is ready for sex...but make no mistake: a few "droops" and she'll bare her teeth!*

According to sextrology, the favorite positions of the Taurus female are 1-3, 11-2, 10-1, 6-2 (not necessarily in that order).
For details, see the chapter on positions.

According to Western Astrology

The relationship between the Taurus male/female and the members of the other signs:

Aries:
A dangerous mixture that can lead to an explosion!

Taurus:
Convenient, predictable, but sometimes yawningly boring...

Gemini:
Each for his own, in life as well as in bed.

Cancer:
A good life, making the most of every moment.

Leo:
Personality contrasts are expressed in every field.

Virgo:
These go well together.

Libra:
Thunder and lightning, for good and for bad.

Scorpio:
Mutual consideration, gentle and pleasurable sex.

According to Western Astrology

Sagittarius:
Differences that are difficult to bridge.

Capricorn:
An interesting combination, full of happy surprises.

Aquarius:
Endless rows that stop only in bed.

Pisces:
An extremely fruitful match.

Sextrology

The aim of this questionnaire is to determine how well the **Taurus man** matches the sextrological profile presented in this book.

Answer only Yes or No for each question. It is mandatory to answer all the questions.

Yes/No 1. Can you react to changing situations in a relationship that involves sex?

Yes/No 2. Do you need a long time before and during sexual arousal?

Yes/No 3. Do you prefer sex - even if it is routine and institutionalized - to a decadent gourmet meal?

Yes/No 4. Is it the opinion of your partner that sex with you is long and drawn-out?

Yes/No 5. Do you prefer the routine to the innovative and the bizarre?

Yes/No 6. Do you have sex - or at least want to have sex - more often than is the norm in your age group?

Yes/No 7. Do you sometimes use sex as a refuge from the troubles of this world?

Add up the positive answers.

If you answered "Yes" to one or two of the questions, you match the profile of the Taurus man "poorly."

If you answered "Yes" to three, four, or five of the questions, you match the profile of the Taurus man "in an average and normal way."

If you answered "Yes" to six or seven of the questions, you match the profile of the Taurus man "well."

Sextrology

Now we will add the questionnaire that the expert in Indian astrology and in the *Kama Sutra* would have constructed:

Do you define yourself as a rabbit, an ox, or a horse?

Now find the category to which you belong by following the simple procedure below:

(1) Circle the category (Rabbit, Ox, or Horse) that describes you.

(2) Circle the category (Poorly, Average & normal, or Well) according to your questionnaire score.

(3) Find the number where the two above categories meet. This number is your sextrological matching number.

	Rabbit	**Ox**	**Horse**
Poorly	1	2	3
Average & normal	4	5	6
Well	7	8	9

Sextrology

The aim of this questionnaire is to determine how well the **Taurus woman** matches the sextrological profile presented in this book.

Answer only Yes or No for each question. It is mandatory to answer all the questions.

Yes/No 1. Would you ever show direct and blunt initiative when going after a man?
Yes/No 2. Do you think that the best place to actualize a sexual relationship is in your bedroom?
Yes/No 3. Do you believe that a man who cheats on you cannot love you?
Yes/No 4. Do you consider the outward expressions of a relationship - courtship, little gifts, phone calls and so on - to be more important than the physical expression?
Yes/No 5. Do you believe that when a man gives you an expensive gift or takes you to a fancy restaurant, he should be rewarded with sex?
Yes/No 6. If you need a long time to reach orgasm, are you afraid that the man won't be up to the task?
Yes/No 7. Do you rush to tell anyone who is prepared to listen that you've got a man who's "yours" and only yours?

Add up the positive answers.

If you answered "Yes" to one or two of the questions, you match the profile of the Taurus woman "poorly."

If you answered "Yes" to three, four, or five of the questions, you match the profile of the Taurus woman "in an average and normal way."

Sextrology

If you answered "Yes" to six or seven of the questions, you match the profile of the Taurus woman "well."

Now we will add the questionnaire that the expert in Indian astrology and in the *Kama Sutra* would have constructed:

Do you define yourself as a deer, a mare, or an elephant?

Now find the category to which you belong by following the simple procedure below:
(1) Circle the category (Deer, Mare, or Elephant) that describes you.
(2) Circle the category (Poorly, Average & normal, or Well) according to you questionnaire score.
(3) Find the number where the two above categories meet. This number is your sextrological matching number.

	Deer	**Mare**	**Elephant**
Poor	1	2	3
Average & normal	4	5	6
Well	7	8	9

According to Western Astrology

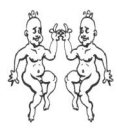

Gemini

Gemini people of both sexes are mainly characterized by their very strong ties to their families - both in love and in sex. The Gemini male or female is inclined to learn his or her sexuality from sisters, cousins, and other family members.

The Gemini male never gives himself entirely. He is a successful lover who does his job with all his heart, but he always maintains a little distance.

His sexual ties are brief, he switches partners frequently, and his marriage tends to land up on the rocks.

The Gemini male is competitive by nature, and is inclined to bring his competitiveness into the bedroom, too. He always tries to be "the best" his partner ever had, and is insulted by any reproachful comment she may make.

The Gemini male marries in order to establish a family, but he does not see his spouse as his equal, always preferring his own family to her and her family.

The Gemini female looks for the image of her father in men. She loves being wooed by many guys, but does not surrender easily. Many Gemini females have earned the nickname "cock-teasers" because they let their partners get really turned on, but don't let them reach orgasm.

The Gemini woman generally loses her virginity to a childhood friend or even a relative, and her sexual experience prior to her marriage will be limited.

According to Western Astrology

After she gets married, the Gemini woman takes care of her home "so it's like Mom's house" and tries to raise her children to have a cordial relationship with the other family members.

The Gemini male

The Gemini male is tall and thin, and if he does not work at physical fitness, his health tends to suffer. His penis is long and thin, and somewhat flaccid.

He sees sexual intercourse as part of a whole scenario - from the moment he meets his partner, he is part of a game of courtship and love, and sex is one of its parts. Intercourse is not the attainment of an extraordinary peak, but rather an almost essential stage in the relationship.

The Gemini male adapts himself to his partner's temperament, and fits in with any position she likes.

Sometimes, the softness of his organ jeopardizes sexual intercourse, and as a result, its full length and potential are not realized.

Important: *The Gemini male is often a turn-on visually, but not from the point of view of his tool.*

According to sextrology, the favorite positions of the Gemini male are 5-1, 1-2, 6-3, 9-1 (not necessarily in that order).
For details, see the chapter on positions.

The Gemini female

The Gemini female spends her life seeking her "other half," the man. If she finds the right guy, her life will be as happy as can be.

Unfortunately, however, if she does not find the right man, she is liable to go into a decline, to "break" spiritually, and even sink into a distressing depression.

The Gemini female is the perfect partner for sex games (even when she is playing around with someone of the same sex). She is always ready, loves every possible variation, but does not get tired of a routine sex life, either.

The Gemini female never deprecate a man who is not equipped to her liking, so long as he knows what to do with what he's got.

In fact, the Gemini female demands to be related to, above and beyond the sexual level, and this is the key to her behavior. She demands that people relate to her, to her personality, talents, and aspirations... and then she will give her body and temperament to the man who is with her.

If she is not related to in the way she wants, she will not unveil her talents and stormy temperament fully in bed.

The Gemini female is prepared to try every type of sexual position, but she always prefers positions in which she can talk to him (the need to talk also prevents her from having to engage in other oral activities).

She sometimes has trouble reaching the first orgasm, but, having reached it, she can come over and over again.

Important: *The Gemini female, as a sex partner, reaches full bloom with a loving husband - generally speaking after the birth of a child!*

According to sextrology, the favorite positions of the Gemini female are 12-1, 7-2, 11-1, 8-1 (not necessarily in that order).
For details, see the chapter on positions.

According to Western Astrology

The relationship between the *Gemini* male/female and the members of the other signs:

Aries:
Mutual fruitfulness.

Taurus:
Each one is only interested in doing his own thing, which is detrimental to their life together.

Gemini:
Never a dull moment... surprises in sex.

Cancer:
Arguments, arguments, arguments... when is there time for anything else?

Leo:
Tolerable.

Virgo:
Arguments about spiritual matters, but total compatibility in bodily matters.

Libra:
Great.

According to Western Astrology

Scorpio:
Watch out. There is a thin border line that must be carefully preserved.

Sagittarius:
Mutual admiration.

Capricorn:
A weak bond, both in and out of bed.

Aquarius:
A spiritual bond that does not always reach physical expression.

Pisces:
Thunder and lightning.

Sextrology

The aim of this questionnaire is to determine how well the **Gemini man** matches the sextrological profile presented in this book.

Answer only Yes or No for each question. It is mandatory to answer all the questions.

Yes/No 1. Do you know and are you prepared to try - at least in theory - a broad range of types of intercourse?

Yes/No 2. Do you have a great deal of knowledge - even if it is not always practical - about sex?

Yes/No 3. Is sex ever just a means of physical release for you?

Yes/No 4. Are you in the habit of having more than one relationship involving sex simultaneously?

Yes/No 5. Is sex in itself important to you, or must your friends and acquaintances also know that you're having sex?

Yes/No 6. Can you forgive a partner who cheated on you?

Yes/No 7. Do you feel that you often don't reach peaks of satisfaction in a sexual relationship?

Add up the positive answers.

If you answered "Yes" to one or two of the questions, you match the profile of the Gemini man "poorly."

If you answered "Yes" to three, four, or five of the questions, you match the profile of the Gemini man "in an average and normal way."

If you answered "Yes" to six or seven of the questions, you match the profile of the Gemini man "well."

Sextrology

Now we will add the questionnaire that the expert in Indian astrology and in the *Kama Sutra* would have constructed:

Do you define yourself as a rabbit, an ox, or a horse?

Now find the category to which you belong by following the simple procedure below:

(1) Circle the category (Rabbit, Ox, or Horse) that describes you.

(2) Circle the category (Poorly, Average & normal, or Well) according to your questionnaire score.

(3) Find the number where the two above categories meet. This number is your sextrological matching number.

	Rabbit	**Ox**	**Horse**
Poorly	1	2	3
Average & normal	4	5	6
Well	7	8	9

Sextrology

The aim of this questionnaire is to determine how well the **Gemini woman** matches the sextrological profile presented in this book.

Answer only Yes or No for each question. It is mandatory to answer all the questions.

Yes/No 1. Do you ever see yourself as the property of the man who is with you?

Yes/No 2. Do you prefer your partner to be less than five years older than you or less than five years younger than you?

Yes/No 3. Do you ever catch yourself thinking about your grocery list or TV programs during intercourse?

Yes/No 4. Would you ever permit your partner to go on vacation without you?

Yes/No 5. If your sex life is not "sublime," do you think it is mainly your partner's fault?

Yes/No 6. Are you prepared to stand at the side of your partner who is perfect in every way, even if the earth doesn't move when you're making love?

Yes/No 7. Do you believe that women cheat on their partners only if they are sexually frustrated?

Add up the positive answers.

If you answered "Yes" to one or two of the questions, you match the profile of the Gemini woman "poorly."

If you answered "Yes" to three, four, or five of the questions, you match the profile of the Gemini woman "in an average and normal way."

If you answered "Yes" to six or seven of the questions, you match the profile of the Gemini woman "well."

Sextrology

Now we will add the questionnaire that the expert in Indian astrology and in the *Kama Sutra* would have constructed:

Do you define yourself as a deer, a mare, or an elephant?

Now find the category to which you belong by following the simple procedure below:
(1) Circle the category (Deer, Mare, or Elephant) that describes you.
(2) Circle the category (Poorly, Average & normal, or Well) according to you questionnaire score.
(3) Find the number where the two above categories meet. This number is your sextrological matching number.

	Deer	**Mare**	**Elephant**
Poor	1	2	3
Average & normal	4	5	6
Well	7	8	9

According to Western Astrology

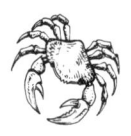

Cancer

Cancer, the crab, who carries his home with him wherever he goes, certainly characterizes the people who bear his name. The main preoccupation of Cancer people is their home and family.

Cancer people of both sexes cultivate long-term bonds, marry late, and maintain stability in their relationships.

In many cases, the Cancer female loses her virginity at a late age, and to the man she eventually marries.

The Cancer male generally loses his virginity in a brothel, or to a girl who is thought to be "easy," but instead of considering it to be a pleasurable memory, he remembers the event as something unpleasant.

The Cancer female tends to be very hesitant in her sexual trysts. She decides on a particular form of sex for herself, and is not inclined to deviate from it. For her, sexual intercourse is connected to giving birth to children. She bonds with her new family (her husband and children), and tends to neglect her ties with her original family.

The Cancer male, being stable and "sure," is considered to be a suitable marriage partner, but a rather boring bed partner. Only after he has completed the courtship-marriage-family cycle at quite a late age does he turn into a real lover.

When one of the couple is a Cancer person, their family is a "model" family - as if the ideal were based on them.

According to Western Astrology

However, as in many other cases, "still waters run deep," and when disputes and rows occur in such a family, they are lengthy and serious, and cause a lot of harm to both parties.

The Cancer male

The crab is a creature that hides in its shell, and so does the Cancer male. He is short, round, and flaccid. Very luckily for him, his penis, even though it is short, is rounded and quite thick, which makes up for its lack of length.

The Cancer male sees sex as part of a whole love scenario - he is gentle and considerate, comes quickly, and does not become erect a second time, unless quite a long time elapses.

By nature, the Cancer male becomes addicted and submits to all the desires of his partner - even her sadistic tendencies. However, more than anything else, the Cancer male prefers to feel secure in the arms of a plump, motherly woman.

Important: *The Cancer male does not engage in a lot of sex, and if he has it frequently during the course of a week, he will take "time off" later.*

According to sextrology, the favorite positions of the Cancer male are 1-3, 5-3, 2-3, 11-3 (not necessarily in that order).
For details, see the chapter on positions.

The Cancer female

What more can be written about the Cancer female, who is known to be the ideal partner for exciting games in bed? She loves virile, well-hung men, and does not only settle for quality - she also wants quantity!

If necessary, she will not hesitate to maintain a stable of handsome "stallions," and even...shhh, don't tell a soul... to participate in group sex, she being at the center!

Ironically, it is precisely this tendency that causes the self-aware Cancer female to distance herself and even abstain from sex. She is afraid that she will not be able to control herself when she succumbs to the pleasures of intercourse, so she distances herself from all possible temptation, for fear of falling victim to a compulsive addiction to sex.

This leads to a situation in which the orgasmic, sexual, and desirable Cancer female presents herself as a "dry iron maiden" - which causes a high level of mental tension.

Sometimes the Cancer female marries a man who knew her as a dried prune, and finds himself with a juicy peach! This change can cause married life to flourish, and prevent any possible crisis.

It is obvious that in many cases, the man cannot keep up (literally) with the change ... and the result is divorce or frequent extramarital affairs.

The Cancer female prefers any form of sex that involves a great deal of strength, bordering on pain. As a spouse or lover, with the right man, she is really perfect.

Important: *As a result of her fear of her rampant sexuality, the Cancer female sometimes imprisons her body and temperament in bonds of coolness and indifference. One must not only know the vessel, but what is inside it!*

According to sextrology, the favorite positions of the Cancer female are 9-2, 2-3, 12-2, 5-3 (not necessarily in that order).
For details, see the chapter on positions.

According to Western Astrology

The relationship between the Cancer male/female and the members of the other signs:

Aries:
Two parallel lines never meet.

Taurus:
Perfect happiness.

Gemini:
Rows, rows, rows.

Cancer:
A quiet, fulfilling life.

Leo:
Differences of opinion. You can't know who'll be on top and who'll be underneath!

Virgo:
Mutual fruitfulness.

Libra:
The perpetual battle about master-slave bonds is not good for the bedroom.

Scorpio:
A creative relationship.

According to Western Astrology

Sagittarius:
Differences that are difficult to bridge.

Capricorn:
Cooperation and mutual admiration.

Aquarius:
Spiritual differences do not make the physical bond easier.

Pisces:
A creative relationship that can only be beneficial.

Sextrology

The aim of this questionnaire is to determine how well the **Cancer man** matches the sextrological profile presented in this book.

Answer only Yes or No for each question. It is mandatory to answer all the questions.

Yes/No 1. Do you tend to express sexual frustrations in anger, tears, or outbursts?

Yes/No 2. Do you devote more thought and effort to courtship, foreplay and the sexual ambiance than you do to the sexual act itself?

Yes/No 3. Do you always prefer to come together with your partner?

Yes/No 4. Are you incapable of maintaining a lengthy relationship with a partner whom you feel you do not satisfy sexually?

Yes/No 5. Do you sometimes - very infrequently - tend to stray and not be faithful to your partner, and have strong guilt feelings about it?

Yes/No 6. Do you have a strong tendency to be sexually turned on as a result of artificial visual stimuli such as pictures or movies?

Yes/No 7. Do you believe that the best thing is to only have sex that comes from love?

Add up the positive answers.

If you answered "Yes" to one or two of the questions, you match the profile of the Cancer man "poorly."

If you answered "Yes" to three, four, or five of the questions, you match the profile of the Cancer man "in an average and normal way."

Sextrology

If you answered "Yes" to six or seven of the questions, you match the profile of the Cancer man "well."

Now we will add the questionnaire that the expert in Indian astrology and in the *Kama Sutra* would have constructed:

Do you define yourself as a rabbit, an ox, or a horse?

Now find the category to which you belong by following the simple procedure below:
(1) Circle the category (Rabbit, Ox, or Horse) that describes you.
(2) Circle the category (Poorly, Average & normal, or Well) according to your questionnaire score.
(3) Find the number where the two above categories meet. This number is your sextrological matching number.

	Rabbit	**Ox**	**Horse**
Poorly	1	2	3
Average & normal	4	5	6
Well	7	8	9

Sextrology

The aim of this questionnaire is to determine how well the **Cancer woman** matches the sextrological profile presented in this book.

Answer only Yes or No for each question. It is mandatory to answer all the questions.

Yes/No 1. Do you believe that the man must protect, nurture, and safeguard his partner?

Yes/No 2. Do you believe that a couple relationship - especially marriage - is meant to last a lifetime?

Yes/No 3. Do you believe that sex is something that is only done at home - that even a hotel, while on vacation with a partner, is not the proper place for sex?

Yes/No 4. Do you believe that every woman has her own sexual style?

Yes/No 5. Do you believe that "it's forbidden to have sex when the children can hear"?

Yes/No 6. Is it true that you will never forget the first time you had sex with a man?

Yes/No 7. Do you believe that the man with you is the "most man" in the world?

Add up the positive answers.

If you answered "Yes" to one or two of the questions, you match the profile of the Cancer woman "poorly."

If you answered "Yes" to three, four, or five of the questions, you match the profile of the Cancer woman "in an average and normal way."

If you answered "Yes" to six or seven of the questions, you match the profile of the Cancer woman "well."

Sextrology

Now we will add the questionnaire that the expert in Indian astrology and in the *Kama Sutra* would have constructed:

Do you define yourself as a deer, a mare, or an elephant?

Now find the category to which you belong by following the simple procedure below:

(1) Circle the category (Deer, Mare, or Elephant) that describes you.

(2) Circle the category (Poorly, Average & normal, or Well) according to you questionnaire score.

(3) Find the number where the two above categories meet. This number is your sextrological matching number.

	Deer	**Mare**	**Elephant**
Poor	1	2	3
Average & normal	4	5	6
Well	7	8	9

According to Western Astrology

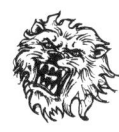

Leo

The lion is the king of the bests, savage and free in the wild.

This is true for the Leo male, too. It is hard to harness him, he shies away from marriage or binding relationships, switches bed partners very frequently, and is considered to be better as a lover than as a marriage partner.

He conquers his partners quickly, takes pride in his conquests, is good in bed... and loves to be complimented about it! When a Leo male loves, his love is incomparably fierce.

When a Leo male is dragged into marriage (and "dragged" is the suitable word), he feels that he is tied down, and plays around extensively. However, if he is faced with the choice of breaking the bonds of matrimony or giving up his cheating, he opts for his marriage.

At a later age, in the third part of life, his sexual prowess declines rapidly, and he devotes his attention to his children or his work instead of women.

The Leo female is generally the "queen of her class" and enjoys the attentions of many admirers - but is always in control of the situation! She tries to stand out in any forum she finds herself in, but also ensures that her reputation remains immaculate.

Although men pursue her, she is the one who "chooses" the man. In sexual relations, she is reserved and maintains

According to Western Astrology

her imposing bearing in bed, too. Having said that, she enjoys sex, and will not forgo it.

The Leo female's behavior occasionally earns her the nickname "refrigerator" - but nothing could be further from the truth! She is aware of her sexual needs and of the proper way to satisfy her needs.

With the right man, the Leo female is a perfect bed partner.

The Leo male

Just as the lion is the animal king, so the Leo male is the bed king. Generally speaking, he is tall and thin, and his penis is long, solid, and quick to become erect. The Leo male is proud of it, and shows it off as much as possible. He considers giving his partner pleasure to be of supreme importance - even more important than his own pleasure - and this property endears him to his sex partners.

The Leo male prefers positions in which he can watch his penis in action. More than anything, he loves to place his partner in front of a wide mirror, stand behind her, and watch the proceedings in the mirror.

The Leo male considers it his obligation to have at least two rounds of victory in each bed.

Despite his excellent qualities, the Leo male is a dangerous bed partner: he is in the habit of boasting about his conquests, and his mouth is as fast as his penis.

Important: *A lion whose mane is clipped is the most dangerous of creatures! It is not advisable to be around when the Leo male becomes a castrated pussy-cat...*

According to sextrology, the favorite positions of the Leo male are 8-2, 9-3, 2-1, 6-1 (not necessarily in that order). For details, see the chapter on positions.

The Leo female

The Leo female was granted a gift that was not given to all women - she is naturally orgasmic, and reaches a climax quickly, with almost every partner. This is why the Leo female engages in sex a lot, to the point of being truly promiscuous. She is aware of her orgasmic capacity, and loves to watch her partner while she is coming, aware of the fact that her pleasure is his pleasure. She is prepared for every sexual variation, especially in the area of foreplay.

Because of her orgasmic capacity, the Leo female can live with almost any man regardless of his prowess or equipment. She is easily satisfied, and if the man is not sufficiently experienced, she will do whatever she has to do in order to reach her climax. Having said that, a passive man, who does not indulge in sex very much, and is not prepared to be "adventurous" - even to a limited extent - will push his partner into other men's beds.

Important: *The Leo female, who is accustomed to a certain standard and amount of sex, is not prepared to forgo quality or quantity. This can lead to crises.*

According to sextrology, the favorite positions of the Leo female are 10-2, 5-1, 6-3, 7-3 (not necessarily in that order).
For details, see the chapter on positions.

According to Western Astrology

The relationship between the *Leo* male/female and the members of the other signs:

Aries:
A life filled with passion.

Taurus:
Differences.

Gemini:
Mutual respect is not always enough.

Cancer:
Different objectives make cooperation difficult.

Leo:
Quarrels all the way.

Virgo:
Nothing special.

Libra:
A combination that has possibilities, but dangers, too.

Scorpio:
It's difficult to match sex that isn't right.

According to Western Astrology

Sagittarius:
A perfect match.

Capricorn:
Opposing aspirations make it difficult for both parties.

Aquarius:
Cooperation and mutual admiration.

Pisces:
A relationship similar to that of the sacrificial victim on the altar and the person who wields the knife.

Sextrology

The aim of this questionnaire is to determine how well the **Leo man** matches the sextrological profile presented in this book.

Answer only Yes or No for each question. It is mandatory to answer all the questions.

Yes/No 1. Is it more important to you what your partner thinks of your exploits in bed than the exploits themselves?

Yes/No 2. Do you feel that you must be better in bed than your present partner's previous man?

Yes/No 3. Are you offended by any criticism of your sexual prowess or equipment?

Yes/No 4. Are you faithful to your partner and does this fidelity lead to great jealousy?

Yes/No 5. Are you not put off by being demonstratively loving in public - to the point that you do not especially care if others can hear or see you when you've having sex?

Yes/No 6. Is your partner's pleasure of cardinal importance to you?

Yes/No 7. Do you prefer having sex with the same partner three times in one night to having sex with three different partners in one night?

Add up the positive answers.

If you answered "Yes" to one or two of the questions, you match the profile of the Leo man "poorly."

If you answered "Yes" to three, four, or five of the questions, you match the profile of the Leo man "in an average and normal way."

Sextrology

If you answered "Yes" to six or seven of the questions, you match the profile of the Leo man "well."

Now we will add the questionnaire that the expert in Indian astrology and in the *Kama Sutra* would have constructed:

Do you define yourself as a rabbit, an ox, or a horse?

Now find the category to which you belong by following the simple procedure below:
(1) Circle the category (Rabbit, Ox, or Horse) that describes you.
(2) Circle the category (Poorly, Average & normal, or Well) according to your questionnaire score.
(3) Find the number where the two above categories meet. This number is your sextrological matching number.

	Rabbit	**Ox**	**Horse**
Poorly	1	2	3
Average & normal	4	5	6
Well	7	8	9

Sextrology

The aim of this questionnaire is to determine how well the **Leo woman** matches the sextrological profile presented in this book.

Answer only Yes or No for each question. It is mandatory to answer all the questions.

Yes/No 1. Do you like to be praised, extolled and adored for your exploits and talents while making love?
Yes/No 2. Do you believe that a man has to be impressive - that is, with status and recognition in society?
Yes/No 3. Do you believe that infidelity is "the end of the world"?
Yes/No 4. Is it true that you are not prepared to look at an erotic book or watch an erotic movie with your partner (even though you'll do it on your own, secretly)?
Yes/No 5. Is it true that tears are both an expression of joy and a demonstration of pain and sorrow for you?
Yes/No 6. Do you think that a woman who has more than two relationships in one year is promiscuous?
Yes/No 7. Do you believe that your mother has no idea of what sex really is?

Add up the positive answers.

If you answered "Yes" to one or two of the questions, you match the profile of the Leo woman "poorly."

If you answered "Yes" to three, four, or five of the questions, you match the profile of the Leo woman "in an average and normal way."

If you answered "Yes" to six or seven of the questions, you match the profile of the Leo woman "well."

Sextrology

Now we will add the questionnaire that the expert in Indian astrology and in the *Kama Sutra* would have constructed:

Do you define yourself as a deer, a mare, or an elephant?

Now find the category to which you belong by following the simple procedure below:
(1) Circle the category (Deer, Mare, or Elephant) that describes you.
(2) Circle the category (Poorly, Average & normal, or Well) according to you questionnaire score.
(3) Find the number where the two above categories meet. This number is your sextrological matching number.

	Deer	**Mare**	**Elephant**
Poor	1	2	3
Average & normal	4	5	6
Well	7	8	9

According to Western Astrology

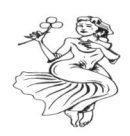

Virgo

Among Virgo people, there is a large gap between sexual character and actual sexual activity.

Regarding Virgo people's sexual character, they "provide for themselves." (Many of them spend their whole lives alone - they do not establish families or have children.)

Virgo people shy away from warm, close relationships, preferring to withdraw into themselves. It is no wonder that their favorite type of sexual activity takes place with the only person they love - in other words, masturbation.

The Virgo female sees a man's shortcomings rather than his good qualities.

She will always remember her first sexual experience - no matter what the actual reality was - as a cruel rape.

She remembers the men with whom she reached orgasm with resentment, because they caused her to lose control of herself.

If the Virgo female marries, she keeps her house clean and respectable, and has a small circle of friends. She takes very little interest in her husband, and will use any excuse to avoid having sex with him.

The Virgo male has striven, since his youth, for solidity and mediocrity in life. This is the case in his studies, his work, his courtship, and his marriage. He is an average lover, does not make much of an impression on his

According to Western Astrology

girlfriends, and is easily hurt by any comment or insinuation about his sexual prowess.

Fortunately, both the Virgo female and male tend to be influenced by other heavenly factors, so only rarely do we find a "pure" Virgo who manifests all the above-mentioned weaknesses.

It's important to remember: Virgo people's sexual ability is far superior to their introverted character!

The Virgo male

The Virgo male is slender in build, average-sized, and physically fit. His penis is average-sized, lacking in girth rather than in length.

However, despite his naive appearance, the Virgo male is well aware of how to make the most of what Nature has given him. After penetrating his partner's heavenly gate, he creates a real commotion, leading to surprises that are not always pleasant.

The Virgo male can prolong intercourse, and when the mood takes him, he can achieve a record-breaking number of erections. He is game for any position, and quickly discovers the one that is most pleasurable for his partner.

Important: *Regarding the Virgo male, don't look at the vessel - look inside it.*

According to sextrology, the favorite positions of the Virgo male are 8-3, 7-1, 6-2, 3-1 (not necessarily in that order). For details, see the chapter on positions.

The Virgo female

If a bunch of Virgo females get together in a room and the conversation revolves around sexual intercourse, the most comprehensive encyclopedia about the topic will emerge! The Virgo female is an endless font of knowledge about sex games and intercourse... everything that females of any other signs know (and do), the Virgo female knows (but doesn't always do) twice and three times as much!

If the Virgo female decides to shift from theory to practice, she is the woman with whom it is possible to have a quickie at a party, stop the car on the way home at the 69th mile, and finish the stormy session at daybreak, with the neighbors banging on the walls in protest at the noises emanating from her apartment... The Virgo female is ready for anything, anywhere - and is always in search of a new trick!

We're not just talking about intercourse. The Virgo female can attain satisfaction from hugging, kissing, or hasty petting, and she doesn't care where - at home, in the car, or at the cinema. She constantly needs a hug, a good word...

And the most amazing thing - the Virgo female is faithful, and devoted to one partner! She will never have a sexual relationship with two men in parallel (or more, of course!).

Sextrology

Moreover - when she leaves the arms of one man, a long period of total celibacy elapses before she lets another man enjoy the pleasures of life.

The Virgo female will do anything to please her man, who will always be the one and only, the best of all. Sex, for her, is a way of pleasing, and not a pursuit of pleasure for its own sake.

Important: *It is advisable for the Virgo female to think ten times before breaking up with the man who is close to her. (If a man breaks up with a Virgo female - knowing exactly what he is losing - he should take a good look in the mirror and try to work out how he took leave of his senses!)*

According to sextrology, the favorite positions of the Virgo female are 8-1, 1-1, 10-3, 6-2 (not necessarily in that order).
For details, see the chapter on positions.

According to Western Astrology

The relationship between the Virgo male/female and the members of the other signs:

Aries:
Master-slave relationship, in sex as well.

Taurus:
A match that promises many pleasures.

Gemini:
A spiritual conflict is not in sync with physical harmony.

Cancer:
Mutual interest, which never hurts.

Leo:
No compatibility, and that's a shame.

Virgo:
Two well-organized cells in one frame.

Libra:
A lack of communication in everyday life as well as in sex.

Scorpio:
Many pleasures.

According to Western Astrology

Sagittarius:
Suffering and sorrow accompanied by a few feelings of happiness.

Capricorn:
Good for marriage, bad for casual affairs.

Aquarius:
Little in common, that sometimes contains a lot.

Pisces:
Contrasts that complement one another.

Sextrology

The aim of this questionnaire is to determine how well the **Virgo man** matches the sextrological profile presented in this book.

Answer only Yes or No for each question. It is mandatory to answer all the questions.

Yes/No 1. Do you think that unless sex is perfect, it's better to forgo it?
Yes/No 2. Is sexual technique more important to you than feeling?
Yes/No 3. Are you suspicious of a partner who tries to get you into bed "too quickly"?
Yes/No 4. Are you suspicious of your partner's "sexual history" to the point of interrogating her about her past?
Yes/No 5. Do you take advantage of when you're having sex to "settle accounts" or release tensions that have accumulated over time?
Yes/No 6. Do you tend to badmouth partners who dumped you?
Yes/No 7. Does it seem to you that your partner is faking her emotions and reactions when she's with you?

Add up the positive answers.

If you answered "Yes" to one or two of the questions, you match the profile of the Virgo man "poorly."

If you answered "Yes" to three, four, or five of the questions, you match the profile of the Virgo man "in an average and normal way."

If you answered "Yes" to six or seven of the questions, you match the profile of the Virgo man "well."

Sextrology

Now we will add the questionnaire that the expert in Indian astrology and in the *Kama Sutra* would have constructed:

Do you define yourself as a rabbit, an ox, or a horse?

Now find the category to which you belong by following the simple procedure below:

(1) Circle the category (Rabbit, Ox, or Horse) that describes you.

(2) Circle the category (Poorly, Average & normal, or Well) according to your questionnaire score.

(3) Find the number where the two above categories meet. This number is your sextrological matching number.

	Rabbit	**Ox**	**Horse**
Poorly	1	2	3
Average & normal	4	5	6
Well	7	8	9

Sextrology

The aim of this questionnaire is to determine how well the **Virgo woman** matches the sextrological profile presented in this book.

Answer only Yes or No for each question. It is mandatory to answer all the questions.

Yes/No 1. Do you believe that sexual satisfaction is the most important thing in a relationship and in life in general?

Yes/No 2. Do you prefer to have sex in the dark, and preferably under the covers?

Yes/No 3. Do you make sure to wash yourself before and immediately after sex?

Yes/No 4. Does talking during sex cool your passion and prevent you from reaching orgasm?

Yes/No 5. In theory, you are prepared to do anything to satisfy your partner. However, do you try to get out of doing something that doesn't give you pleasure?

Yes/No 6. You don't have any criticism of your partner's actions in bed. But do you have a very long list of his faults in your memory?

Yes/No 7. Do you believe that a bird in the hand is better than two in the bush?

Add up the positive answers.

If you answered "Yes" to one or two of the questions, you match the profile of the Virgo woman "poorly."

If you answered "Yes" to three, four, or five of the questions, you match the profile of the Virgo woman "in an average and normal way."

Sextrology

If you answered "Yes" to six or seven of the questions, you match the profile of the Virgo woman "well."

Now we will add the questionnaire that the expert in Indian astrology and in the *Kama Sutra* would have constructed:

Do you define yourself as a deer, a mare, or an elephant?

Now find the category to which you belong by following the simple procedure below:
(1) Circle the category (Deer, Mare, or Elephant) that describes you.
(2) Circle the category (Poorly, Average & normal, or Well) according to you questionnaire score.
(3) Find the number where the two above categories meet. This number is your sextrological matching number.

	Deer	**Mare**	**Elephant**
Poor	1	2	3
Average & normal	4	5	6
Well	7	8	9

According to Western Astrology

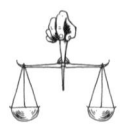

Libra

The Libra female is almost incapable of being without a partner, and when she does not find a suitable one, she chooses one that does not suit her - or even a female partner. Loneliness is the greatest danger for her.

Libra people are quick to establish social ties, have a broad circle of acquaintances, marry quickly and divorce quickly, and are never alone. Libra people adapt themselves to their partner, especially in sexual relations. The Libra female will take part in any sex game her partner desires, and will try to enjoy it. This makes Libra people very popular, and increases their circle of friends.

Libra people are similar, to a great extent, to a creeper that adapts itself to the tree-trunk it is growing on... however, the passage from tree-trunk to tree-trunk is rapid, and Libra people are capable of adapting to almost every tree-trunk!

This adaptive ability is helpful in establishing normal family ties. Libra people nurture their family ties, or other ties, so long as it is pleasant and satisfying for them. The moment there are any hitches, they do not hesitate to break off the relationship and start another one.

Libra people are ideal partners for relationships that are limited in time. The relationship will be pleasant and convenient for its duration, and the separation will be painless.

The Libra male

The Libra male resembles his name - he is well balanced. He is well proportioned, and is a handsome and eye-catching man. His penis is not especially big, but is esthetic, proportionate, and attractive in color.

He considers physical love to be almost a way of life, and from this point of view is a perfect lover. He lingers over foreplay, remains calm during intercourse, knows all the tricks in bed, and is aware of the extensive variety of female sexuality. He always adapts himself to the properties and character of his partner.

The Libra male likes novelty in sex, and seeks out new and varied experiences, either with his partner or without her.

Important: *The Libra male, who loves perfection, is liable to reach a situation in which he favors the one he loves the most - himself. What a shame.*

According to sextrology, the favorite positions of the Libra male are 7-2, 8-1, 10-2, 3-2 (not necessarily in that order).
For details, see the chapter on positions.

The Libra female

The Libra female is somewhat two-faced in her attitude to intercourse and sexual relations. She is not particularly active in anything concerning love games - she prefers to sprawl out on her back and let the man do the work.

For her, sex is a sacred obligation, and when she feels the man's tool penetrating her body, she knows that she has fulfilled her obligation...

And then every changes!

The Libra female, at the point of penetration, reveals the other side of her temperament - she is swept away by the lovemaking, reaches a powerful and noisy orgasm accompanied by thunder and lightning, and occasionally astounds her partner with this unfamiliar and unexpected reaction!

This is what the Libra female is like, and this is what is said about her: "If you haven't made love to a Libra female, you don't know what a woman is!"

Initially, she is indifferent, withdrawn, submissive... and then she becomes a volcano of passion. And if she repeats the act an hour later, her partner will go down the same road again - from indifference to the jet of boiling lava!

Regarding her range of positions and sexual rhythm, the Libra female is not particularly outstanding - but she compensates herself, and her partner, with a tremendous, noisy, and prolonged orgasm.

As we say, "All's well that ends well."

Important: *The Libra female is well advised not to entertain a man in an apartment with thin walls...*

According to sextrology, the favorite positions of the Libra female are 10-2, 11-3, 12-2, 6-1 (not necessarily in that order). For details, see the chapter on positions.

According to Western Astrology

The relationship between the Libra male/female and the members of the other signs:

Aries:
Mutual respect.

Taurus:
An undesirable mixture, whose ingredients are repulsive to one another.

Gemini:
A good match in the correct proportion and at the right time.

Cancer:
Struggle for control.

Leo:
A match in which everything is predictable and the choice is pre-ordained.

Virgo:
A lack of communication is detrimental to sexual performance.

Libra:
Lovely.

According to Western Astrology

Scorpio:
A dangerous match, which has earned the nickname, "The Beauty and the Beast," because of the sexual image.

Sagittarius:
Good for the short term, but fatal in the long term.

Capricorn:
The mutual pursuit of pleasure sometimes comes at the expense of family life.

Aquarius:
A happy couple.

Pisces:
Tension; each party feels like a victim.

Sextrology

The aim of this questionnaire is to determine how well the **Libra man** matches the sextrological profile presented in this book.

Answer only Yes or No for each question. It is mandatory to answer all the questions.

Yes/No 1. Are you better at talking about and describing sex than participating in it?

Yes/No 2. Does your partner think that you're a perfect lover?

Yes/No 3. Do you still remember and regret sex that you missed out on long ago?

Yes/No 4. Do you want to hear about your partner's past sexual relationships?

Yes/No 5. You like sex, but are there many things you like more?

Yes/No 6. Do you believe that "if my partner doesn't come, it's her fault!"?

Yes/No 7. Do you believe that with a suitable partner, sex will be the best thing in the world?

Add up the positive answers.

If you answered "Yes" to one or two of the questions, you match the profile of the Libra man "poorly."

If you answered "Yes" to three, four, or five of the questions, you match the profile of the Libra man "in an average and normal way."

If you answered "Yes" to six or seven of the questions, you match the profile of the Libra man "well."

Sextrology

Now we will add the questionnaire that the expert in Indian astrology and in the *Kama Sutra* would have constructed:

Do you define yourself as a rabbit, an ox, or a horse?

Now find the category to which you belong by following the simple procedure below:

(1) Circle the category (Rabbit, Ox, or Horse) that describes you.
(2) Circle the category (Poorly, Average & normal, or Well) according to your questionnaire score.
(3) Find the number where the two above categories meet. This number is your sextrological matching number.

	Rabbit	**Ox**	**Horse**
Poorly	1	2	3
Average & normal	4	5	6
Well	7	8	9

Sextrology

The aim of this questionnaire is to determine how well the **Libra woman** matches the sextrological profile presented in this book.

Answer only Yes or No for each question. It is mandatory to answer all the questions.

Yes/No 1. Do you believe that your partner showing his emotions is just as important as physical expressions of sexuality?

Yes/No 2. When you want to "guide" your partner to behave as you want him to, can you talk to him for hours?

Yes/No 3. Are your partner's good looks and standing (as well as his home, clothing, and car) more important to you than anything?

Yes/No 4. Do you think that if sex is not good, it's your partner's fault?

Yes/No 5. Is it true that you don't care if your partner holds your hand tightly during sex, but you are not prepared for him to block your mouth?

Yes/No 6. Is it true that you are prepared to share sexual experiences with your girlfriends, but you only tell them about the positive things?

Yes/No 7. When your partner has offended you, are you unable to reach orgasm?

Add up the positive answers.

If you answered "Yes" to one or two of the questions, you match the profile of the Libra woman "poorly."

If you answered "Yes" to three, four, or five of the

questions, you match the profile of the Libra woman "in an average and normal way."

If you answered "Yes" to six or seven of the questions, you match the profile of the Libra woman "well."

Now we will add the questionnaire that the expert in Indian astrology and in the *Kama Sutra* would have constructed:

Do you define yourself as a deer, a mare, or an elephant?

Now find the category to which you belong by following the simple procedure below:

(1) Circle the category (Deer, Mare, or Elephant) that describes you.

(2) Circle the category (Poorly, Average & normal, or Well) according to you questionnaire score.

(3) Find the number where the two above categories meet. This number is your sextrological matching number.

	Deer	**Mare**	**Elephant**
Poor	1	2	3
Average & normal	4	5	6
Well	7	8	9

According to Western Astrology

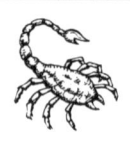

Scorpio

The sign of Scorpio - and we must not forget this - is the sign that projects directly onto the genitals of both male and female. Therefore, the lives of Scorpio people are affected more than anything by their conduct on the sexual level - for good and for bad.

From childhood, Scorpio people exude sexuality. The Scorpio female performs enough sexual experimentation in her youth to last all the women from other signs their entire lives! The Scorpio male gets involved in sexual liaisons with older women.

Just as Scorpio people are attracted to the opposite sex (only a few of them have homosexual or lesbian tendencies), so others are attracted to them. They radiate sexuality.

The Scorpio female is a girl with "come hither" eyes. The Scorpio male is the man who is always ready to leap into bed...

And in that respect, fortunately, the Scorpio male does not let anyone down. He is a perfect lover who never says "I'm beat!"

The Scorpio woman tends to quickly transform the ties she has established with admirers into bedroom relationships. While she is very responsive to being courted, she never submits, but is always an equal partner with her own rights in bed.

According to Western Astrology

The focus on sexual relations only rarely contributes to the stability of the Scorpio male's family life - only if he finds a partner who understands and fits in with his tendencies will he find peace at home. In general, Scorpio men are champions at playing around.

The Scorpio female, too, who is well aware of the pleasures of sex, would happily sacrifice a little of her morality in order to relive her youthful experiences.

Sextrology

The Scorpio male

The scorpion is ready to sting anything at any given moment, and so is the Scorpio male. Regardless of his appearance, he is always ready for battle. His penis - regardless of its size - becomes erect in an instant. Some people claim that even the thought of a shapely leg is enough to turn the Scorpio male on!

The Scorpio male is proud of his penis and takes full advantage of it. Sexual intercourse with a Scorpio male resembles a long battle consisting of thrusts and penetrations. More than anything, he loves using his organ like a pestle in a mortar, and revels in doing this for amazing lengths of time, for his partner's enjoyment.

This mechanical action is liable to become boring and tiresome after some time... but until then, the results are extremely pleasurable.

Important: *The Scorpio male is so enchanted by the perpetual in-out motion of his penis that he sometimes forgets all the rest.*

According to sextrology, the favorite positions of the Scorpio male are 4-2, 1-2, 11-2, 12-2 (not necessarily in that order).
For details, see the chapter on positions.

The Scorpio female

What more can be added to the glory of the Scorpio female?

In many cases, the Scorpio female is synonymous with "nymphomaniac"! Only ignorant people would perceive her like that, however; the Scorpio female is blessed with an abundantly sexual temperament.

Period.

The Scorpio female likes men, and loves to examine the extent of manliness hidden in every pair of pants that shows up. She is prepared to try each one out...and then she finds out for herself which the best of the bunch are, and discards the ones that failed the test. Many women are prepared to settle for the leftovers from the Scorpio female's bed...

Virile, well-hung, and very fit guys are suitable partners for the Scorpio female. She uses her body to test-drive them, investigates the limits of their abilities, and gives grades (very meticulously, to their regret!).

The Scorpio female often keeps one man at her side, but she does not forgo her forays into other beds. She has more than enough to give to more than one man.

Although she has lots of men, her love is given to only one. She differentiates perfectly well between an act of intercourse and an act of love.

The Scorpio female loves fast, rough intercourse, even if it does not go on for long.

Important: *The Scorpio female loves sexual intercourse as a physical and emotional need, and sometimes this love of sex turns into a way of life for her - never as a "professional," however, who takes money for her services.*

According to sextrology, the favorite positions of the Scorpio female are 7-3, 9-3, 5-2, 8-2 (not necessarily in that order).
For details, see the chapter on positions.

According to Western Astrology

The relationship between the Scorpio male/female and the members of the other signs:

Aries:
Too many rows and arguments.

Taurus:
Mutual consideration.

Gemini:
A fine border, beyond which there is an abyss of rows and arguments.

Cancer:
A great relationship, from all points of view.

Leo:
Each one pulls in his own direction.

Virgo:
Practical, fulfills itself.

Libra:
A relationship that is reminiscent of "The Beauty and the Beast."

Scorpio:
All the possibilities are offered - happiness or suffering.

According to Western Astrology

Sagittarius:
They each safeguard their own uniqueness.

Capricorn:
A match filled with happiness for the couple and their immediate surroundings.

Aquarius:
Opposing aims.

Pisces:
The members of the couple adapt to each other.

Sextrology

The aim of this questionnaire is to determine how well the **Scorpio man** matches the sextrological profile presented in this book.

Answer only Yes or No for each question. It is mandatory to answer all the questions.

Yes/No 1. Do you believe that the ideal thing is emotion that leads to love that leads to sex?

Yes/No 2. Do you believe that quality is more important than quantity in sex?

Yes/No 3. If your partner displays sexual knowledge and expertise that is "out of the ordinary," do you begin to doubt her decency and morality?

Yes/No 4. "I'll never get into a relationship with a woman who has stripped in public!" Is that your opinion?

Yes/No 5. Do you believe that it is better for partners to sleep in separate beds or separate rooms, and not in a double bed?

Yes/No 6. Do you want everyone to know how much you love your partner and how much she loves you?

Yes/No 7. Is it true that you would never perform a sexual act under duress, or without the explicit consent of your partner?

Add up the positive answers.

If you answered "Yes" to one or two of the questions, you match the profile of the Scorpio man "poorly."

If you answered "Yes" to three, four, or five of the questions, you match the profile of the Scorpio man "in an average and normal way."

Sextrology

If you answered "Yes" to six or seven of the questions, you match the profile of the Scorpio man "well."

Now we will add the questionnaire that the expert in Indian astrology and in the *Kama Sutra* would have constructed:

Do you define yourself as a rabbit, an ox, or a horse?

Now find the category to which you belong by following the simple procedure below:

(1) Circle the category (Rabbit, Ox, or Horse) that describes you.

(2) Circle the category (Poorly, Average & normal, or Well) according to your questionnaire score.

(3) Find the number where the two above categories meet. This number is your sextrological matching number.

	Rabbit	**Ox**	**Horse**
Poorly	1	2	3
Average & normal	4	5	6
Well	7	8	9

Sextrology

The aim of this questionnaire is to determine how well the **Scorpio woman** matches the sextrological profile presented in this book.

Answer only Yes or No for each question. It is mandatory to answer all the questions.

Yes/No 1. When you don't have sex as much as you're used to, do you feel that you're "climbing the walls"?

Yes/No 2. Do you believe that extreme jealousy and sometimes even violence on the part of your partner attest to his great love for you?

Yes/No 3. Are you prepared to try anything, cheat, or have several relationships at the same time, as long as you get enjoyment out of it?

Yes/No 4. Do you display a tendency - at least in theory - to have sex in exotic places (on the beach, for instance)?

Yes/No 5. Do you believe that your man must be "stronger" than you?

Yes/No 6. Do you believe that every woman is capable of multiple orgasms, at least in theory?

Yes/No 7. Do you believe that the source of conflicts or divorce always lies in sexual problems?

Add up the positive answers.

If you answered "Yes" to one or two of the questions, you match the profile of the Scorpio woman "poorly."

If you answered "Yes" to three, four, or five of the questions, you match the profile of the Scorpio woman "in an average and normal way."

Sextrology

If you answered "Yes" to six or seven of the questions, you match the profile of the Scorpio woman "well."

Now we will add the questionnaire that the expert in Indian astrology and in the Kama Sutra would have constructed:

Do you define yourself as a deer, a mare, or an elephant?

Now find the category to which you belong by following the simple procedure below:
(1) Circle the category (Deer, Mare, or Elephant) that describes you.
(2) Circle the category (Poorly, Average & normal, or Well) according to you questionnaire score.
(3) Find the number where the two above categories meet. This number is your sextrological matching number.

	Deer	**Mare**	**Elephant**
Poor	1	2	3
Average & normal	4	5	6
Well	7	8	9

According to Western Astrology

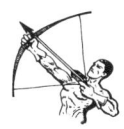

Sagittarius

The Sagittarius person, like the Virgo person, provides for himself. However, unlike the Virgo person, the Sagittarius person does not withdraw into himself, but rather is open to the world, congenial, and gregarious.

These properties make him the perfect lover - he defends his independence, and also gives of himself with all his heart.

Defending his independence enables the Sagittarius male to share his love with many women - simultaneously. He gives all of himself to all of them.

This quality is also conspicuous in the Sagittarius female, and for this reason, anyone who is married to a Sagittarius person must be aware of this dichotomy.

The Sagittarius female can leave her home and her family at the drop of a hat and follow her lover (the Sagittarius male does not tend to do this for fear of making a new commitment that will limit his independence.)

The lives of Sagittarius people of both sexes are not stable. Home and family are not at the top of their list of priorities.

While they are charming partners and guests at every party, and all their friends have nothing but good things to say about them, their personal, inner lives lack stability.

The Sagittarius male

The Sagittarius male has a penis that is reminiscent of an arrow in a bow - long and protruding, with a fat belly above it. He is characterized by the combination of a handsome penis, a paunch, and poor physical fitness.

He likes sexual intercourse, but is aware of his limitations - he prefers brief sex in which he does not have to move a lot or vigorously, but having said that, takes full advantage of his penis.

The Sagittarius male, aware of his limitations, is quite a good lover, and will generally go for a second round after a suitable period of rest.

Unfortunately, his poor physical condition jeopardizes his sexual activity at a later age.

Important: Don't wear the Sagittarius male out before he fires - he may not have the strength to draw his bow and shoot his arrow.

According to sextrology, the favorite positions of the Sagittarius male are 5-1, 1-1, 4-1, 11-1 (not necessarily in that order).
For details, see the chapter on positions.

The Sagittarius female

The Sagittarius female combines the sexuality of the Leo female and the lust of the Scorpio female. Her exceptional ability to reach orgasm anywhere, anyhow, and with anyone, together with her passion for the pleasures of sex, make her into the perfect partner for quick rolls in the hay, the focal point of every party... and the perfect partner for horny men.

The Sagittarius female is naive, to a certain extent - she can begin an evening with a friendly hug and an hour later find herself sprawled on her back, skirt around her waist! She does not see anything reprehensible about this... and the fact is that even a chance roll in the hay brings her to orgasm and satisfies her... for the next hour, at least!

The Sagittarius female loves being gratifying by the man's fingers, mouth, and tongue, perhaps because she is afraid that the man will not be able to withstand her sexual demands over any length of time.

During intercourse, she gives herself totally to the man, but she is not "easy" by nature. A Sagittarius female who lives with a man who satisfies her sexuality will never cheat on him, even if his virility cannot satisfy her demands.

In general, she prefers not to "bombard" the man with too many sexual acts, and gives him the pleasure of satisfying her with "love toys" in the sex game.

Sextrology

The Sagittarius female has a natural capacity for multiple orgasms, and exudes warmth and love on the man or men with her.

The moment the compatibility between her and her partner deteriorates, she prefers to break up with him rather than cheat on him. In many cases, she will use her hands to help the man become virile again, and prefers masturbation to infidelity.

Important: *The Sagittarius female must not just be judged according to the ease with which she gives herself - she does not use sex as bait! It is a deep and natural need of her body!*

According to sextrology, the favorite positions of the Sagittarius female are 2-1, 3-2, 9-1, 4-2 (not necessarily in that order).
For details, see the chapter on positions.

According to Western Astrology

The relationship between the Sagittarius male/female and the members of the other signs:

Aries:
Happy together.

Taurus:
Differences that cause conflicts.

Gemini:
Mutual admiration that overcomes any possible misgivings about each other.

Cancer:
Parallel lines don't meet.

Leo:
A match that is full of happiness and enjoyable activity.

Virgo:
Tension, rows, and disputes.

Libra:
Perfect harmony.

Scorpio:
A mixture whose components remain forever.

According to Western Astrology

Sagittarius:
A good match for casual encounters.

Capricorn:
Different temperaments lead to a collision in everyday life.

Aquarius:
A happy affair, just like in the movies.

Pisces:
Better in spirit than in body.

Sextrology

The aim of this questionnaire is to determine how well the **Sagittarius man** matches the sextrological profile presented in this book.

Answer only Yes or No for each question. It is mandatory to answer all the questions.

Yes/No 1. Are you ready for sexual activity at any time, in any situation, and with any woman?

Yes/No 2. Do you use sex as a means of punishing or rewarding your partner?

Yes/No 3. Do you believe that sex is meant first and foremost to satisfy your lust?

Yes/No 4. Is it true that nothing holds you back when you're courting a new partner?

Yes/No 5. Do you occasionally find yourself hurt, or paying dearly, for your various sexual addictions?

Yes/No 6. Do you believe that your daughters must refrain from any contact with men?

Yes/No 7. Are you always prepared - at least in theory - to let another woman join you and your partner in bed, but if your partner as much as hinted at bringing another man into your bed, you would break up with her?

Add up the positive answers.

If you answered "Yes" to one or two of the questions, you match the profile of the Sagittarius man "poorly."

If you answered "Yes" to three, four, or five of the questions, you match the profile of the Sagittarius man "in an average and normal way."

Sextrology

If you answered "Yes" to six or seven of the questions, you match the profile of the Sagittarius man "well."

Now we will add the questionnaire that the expert in Indian astrology and in the *Kama Sutra* would have constructed:

Do you define yourself as a rabbit, an ox, or a horse?

Now find the category to which you belong by following the simple procedure below:

(1) Circle the category (Rabbit, Ox, or Horse) that describes you.
(2) Circle the category (Poorly, Average & normal, or Well) according to your questionnaire score.
(3) Find the number where the two above categories meet. This number is your sextrological matching number.

	Rabbit	**Ox**	**Horse**
Poorly	1	2	3
Average & normal	4	5	6
Well	7	8	9

Sextrology

The aim of this questionnaire is to determine how well the **Sagittarius woman** matches the sextrological profile presented in this book.

Answer only Yes or No for each question. It is mandatory to answer all the questions.

Yes/No 1. Do you believe that it's your right to try anything?

Yes/No 2. Do you believe that being in a relationship need not stop you from seeing what's going on around you - in other words, you can look in store windows, even if you do the shopping at home?

Yes/No 3. In your opinion, are courtship, foreplay, and little gifts just as important to the relationship as sex itself?

Yes/No 4. Does the expression, "I'm not prepared to play by the rules," reflect your outlook?

Yes/No 5. There are things you are amazingly stubborn about. For instance, if your partner asked you to shave your legs, would you do it?

Yes/No 6. Do you believe that failures and crises in a sexual relationship are natural, and do not constitute a reason for breaking up?

Yes/No 7. Do you believe that what someone don't know won't hurt him?

Add up the positive answers.

If you answered "Yes" to one or two of the questions, you match the profile of the Sagittarius woman "poorly."

If you answered "Yes" to three, four, or five of the

Sextrology

questions, you match the profile of the Sagittarius woman "in an average and normal way."

If you answered "Yes" to six or seven of the questions, you match the profile of the Sagittarius woman "well."

Now we will add the questionnaire that the expert in Indian astrology and in the *Kama Sutra* would have constructed:

Do you define yourself as a deer, a mare, or an elephant?

Now find the category to which you belong by following the simple procedure below:

(1) Circle the category (Deer, Mare, or Elephant) that describes you.

(2) Circle the category (Poorly, Average & normal, or Well) according to you questionnaire score.

(3) Find the number where the two above categories meet. This number is your sextrological matching number.

	Deer	**Mare**	**Elephant**
Poor	1	2	3
Average & normal	4	5	6
Well	7	8	9

According to Western Astrology

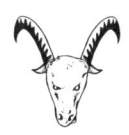

Capricorn

The Capricorn male is sober and calculated in all his actions, and considers every social tie he establishes to be an increase or a decrease in the status he has acquired. He will not get embroiled in an affair on the side, not because he doesn't want to, but because he is afraid that it will cause a scandal. He marries the "right" girl and tries to do right by her.

The Capricorn female is even more calculated in her actions than the male.

She already starts thinking about marriage at a young age, and when she has selected her target, focuses all her attention on her chosen man.

The Capricorn female is moral - not just outwardly, but also within herself - and there is no pretence about her morality.

Capricorn people of both sexes meticulously fulfill their obligations to the public and to their families, and also consider engaging in enjoyable sex to be an "obligation" - which is sometimes detrimental to their sexual relationships.

Capricorn people are honest in their relationships; generally speaking, they don't deceive their partners, and they don't cavort in strange beds.

The Capricorn male, because of the feeling of obligation and the cool-headedness of his deeds, is conservative in his

According to Western Astrology

thoughts, which leads to conflicts with his children - especially with his daughters.

The Capricorn male and female are the most stable of the signs of the Zodiac, and this stability radiates from them onto their partners (who belong to other signs), too. Their sense of obligation is beneficial to society as a whole, and they are central to the entire structure of society.

The Capricorn male

The Capricorn male is really a goat in bed. He is thin and fit, and has a large and erect penis, which knows exactly when to stand to attention. The Capricorn male does not disappoint his partner in bed, no matter whatever her demands may be.

He moves a lot, is mischievous, and uses his hands and mouth during the entire sexual act. By nature, he prefers one high-quality session a week to daily trysts.

The Capricorn male belongs to a sign that tends to fight urges, and it is possible to find males of this sign with not unappreciable talents who favor a life of celibacy and calm over a life spent pursuing the pleasures of the flesh.

Important: *The Capricorn male does not like comparisons, especially not with men who are better endowed than he is!*

According to sextrology, the favorite positions of the Capricorn male are 12-1, 10-1, 2-2, 10-3 (not necessarily in that order).
For details, see the chapter on positions.

The Capricorn female

The Capricorn female learned that "the rope goes after the bucket" - for her, love is the center of life. If she falls in love with somebody (male or female), she will rush to jump into bed with him, learn to fulfill his desires, and adapt herself to his sexual technique.

Without love, there is almost no chance of finding a Capricorn female in any man's bed!

The Capricorn female's disappointment is as great as her love. Her heartbreaks are serious. She sinks into a long period of heartache, depression, and crisis, and quite clearly sex is not at the top of her list of priorities.

It can be said that the Capricorn female considers sex to be the completion of love - she enjoys intercourse, even though she does not always reach breathtaking orgasms. She will not jump into a man's bed just for a roll in the hay, or to win his heart.

No! With her, there has to be love before she spreads her legs...

During the periods between "great" loves, the Capricorn female settles for heart-to-heart conversations with her girl friends, and, if necessary, self-gratification.

The emphasis on love makes the Capricorn female a partner suitable for men who are not particularly hot-blooded. A Capricorn female who has reached a stable,

Sextrology

ongoing relationship with her "great love" will make every effort to see that the flame is not extinguished. Some people claim that there is nothing like a Capricorn female to rouse the sleeping penis!

Important: *The Capricorn female is easily seduced by smooth talk, false promises, and oversights on the way to the great love. She must examine the "great love" under a microscope before making her way to his bed.*

According to sextrology, the favorite positions of the Capricorn female are 1-3, 2-1, 4-3, 3-3 (not necessarily in that order).
For details, see the chapter on positions.

According to Western Astrology

The relationship between the Capricorn male/female and the members of the other signs:

Aries:
Contrasts in personalities.

Taurus:
A happy match.

Gemini:
A weak relationship, devoid of contact and lacking in real enthusiasm.

Cancer:
Fit together like a mortar and pestle.

Leo:
Opposing ambitions are not beneficial.

Virgo:
A perfect couple for marriage.

Libra:
The pursuit of pleasure overcomes any other consideration.

Scorpio:
Happy in each other's arms.

According to Western Astrology

Sagittarius:
It's difficult to mix oil and water...

Capricorn:
A stable, long-term relationship.

Aquarius:
A relationship that doesn't materialize often.

Pisces:
Lovely!

Sextrology

The aim of this questionnaire is to determine how well the **Capricorn man** matches the sextrological profile presented in this book.

Answer only Yes or No for each question. It is mandatory to answer all the questions.

Yes/No   1. Do you differentiate between love that is linked to emotion and sex that is linked to the body?

Yes/No   2. Can you have close relationships with women without having sex with them?

Yes/No   3. Do you feel that the longer a relationship continues, the less pleasurable sex becomes?

Yes/No   4. Do you believe that you could never love and remain in a relationship with a partner who does not satisfy your desires in bed?

Yes/No   5. Is it true that your desire to "rush and tell the guys" is as strong as your sexual urge?

Yes/No   6. Is it true that you remember every failure, every "oops!" in sex, but you don't remember the "successes" and the highs?

Yes/No   7. In your opinion, is it OK for men to cheat on their partners, but it's a no-no for women to cheat on theirs?

Add up the positive answers.

If you answered "Yes" to one or two of the questions, you match the profile of the Capricorn man "poorly."

If you answered "Yes" to three, four, or five of the questions, you match the profile of the Capricorn man "in an average and normal way."

Sextrology

If you answered "Yes" to six or seven of the questions, you match the profile of the Capricorn man "well."

Now we will add the questionnaire that the expert in Indian astrology and in the *Kama Sutra* would have constructed:

Do you define yourself as a rabbit, an ox, or a horse?

Now find the category to which you belong by following the simple procedure below:

(1) Circle the category (Rabbit, Ox, or Horse) that describes you.
(2) Circle the category (Poorly, Average & normal, or Well) according to your questionnaire score.
(3) Find the number where the two above categories meet. This number is your sextrological matching number.

	Rabbit	**Ox**	**Horse**
Poorly	1	2	3
Average & normal	4	5	6
Well	7	8	9

Sextrology

The aim of this questionnaire is to determine how well the **Capricorn woman** matches the sextrological profile presented in this book.

Answer only Yes or No for each question. It is mandatory to answer all the questions.

Yes/No 1. Is it true that you would never go to bed with a man on the first date?

Yes/No 2. Do you believe that it is the man's job to determine the couple's sexual pace or sexual technique?

Yes/No 3. Is it true that you are prepared to do anything for your man - so long as he loves you and is faithful to you?

Yes/No 4. Do you think that only promiscuous women talk about their sexual exploits in public?

Yes/No 5. Is it true that you could never feel comfortable with a former lover... especially when your current lover is also present?

Yes/No 6. Do you believe that there is no way back after divorce?

Yes/No 7. Do you believe that the frequency of sex represents the strength of the relationship - the more often sex occurs, the stronger the relationship?

Add up the positive answers.

If you answered "Yes" to one or two of the questions, you match the profile of the Capricorn woman "poorly."

If you answered "Yes" to three, four, or five of the questions, you match the profile of the Capricorn woman "in an average and normal way."

Sextrology

If you answered "Yes" to six or seven of the questions, you match the profile of the Capricorn woman "well."

Now we will add the questionnaire that the expert in Indian astrology and in the *Kama Sutra* would have constructed:

Do you define yourself as a deer, a mare, or an elephant?

Now find the category to which you belong by following the simple procedure below:
(1) Circle the category (Deer, Mare, or Elephant) that describes you.
(2) Circle the category (Poorly, Average & normal, or Well) according to you questionnaire score.
(3) Find the number where the two above categories meet. This number is your sextrological matching number.

	Deer	**Mare**	**Elephant**
Poor	1	2	3
Average & normal	4	5	6
Well	7	8	9

According to Western Astrology

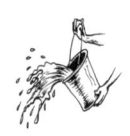

Aquarius

Aquarius males and females are slightly peculiar in their attitude toward love and sex - outwardly, they are cool, withdrawn, and quiet... but after the barriers have come down, they reveal themselves to be extremely potent, warm, and loving lovers!

Indeed, the saying, "Still waters run deep," suits Aquarius people to a T.

The Aquarius male does not establish sexual liaisons with people who belong to his own social class - he prefers to do so with a woman who is inferior or superior to him on the social ladder, but not one of his own status. However, after the relationship has begun, he will relate to his partner as his complete equal.

The Aquarius female prefers people who belong to her own social class. She is a girl with whom all her classmates are friends, and after her marriage, she will carry on her little affairs with friends....

With Aquarius people, life's events are generally inevitable - both marriage and infidelities are kind of "forced" on them. However, after these things are "forced" on them, Aquarius people discover that they rather enjoy them.

The Aquarius male is the perfect lover for the woman who wants discretion and secrecy.

Sextrology

The Aquarius male

Aquarius males have always been the most erotic lovers in any bedroom. Regardless of their handsome appearance, physical fitness, or penis, they have always known how to get the most out of themselves and their partners. The sentence that Aquarius males hear most frequently in bed is "Wow! I didn't know it could be so good!"

The Aquarius male loves investigating sexuality in the same way as a chemist loves his test-tubes. He experiments with new techniques, and tries to implement everything he has learned with his partner. He does not rush, and takes his time in intercourse. He loves foreplay and afterplay. He tries to improve every position, and his partner will discover sources of pleasure that her body has never known. It can be said about the Aquarius male that "you don't know what you haven't tried." He is full of surprises, most of them good.

Important: *The Aquarius male, with all good intentions, is capable of using his partners as guinea pigs in his sexual experiments. Not all the guinea pigs like that...*

According to sextrology, the favorite positions of the Aquarius male are 3-2, 12-3, 7-3, 9-2 (not necessarily in that order).
For details, see the chapter on positions.

The Aquarius female

To a certain extent, the Aquarius female is the opposite of the Sagittarius female.

She can enjoy good sex, and reach orgasm, but will never consider intercourse as "just a roll in the hay," and will never be tempted to take off her panties as a favor to any man.

Although her sexual emotions bubble with passion and abandon, she holds herself back amazingly... Even at her moment of climax, she is careful not to let the expression of self-respect and self-importance on her face disappear! She never screams or writhes, and certainly never scratches her partner!

With her, sex is paced and planned, as is the respectable position in which she places herself.

The Aquarius female determines her schedule for sexual intercourse, always with a carefully chosen partner with whom she has other ties besides sex - be it her husband, her boss, or her first-floor neighbor!

The Aquarius female halts her emotions during intercourse. If she has established a steady relationship with a man, she will have less and less sex with him over the years, and then it will mainly be in order to "do her duty."

Only infrequently will the Aquarius female be swept into

a stormy sexual relationship (which will ultimately lead to the destruction of other relationships in her life).

The Aquarius female usually finds her partner by emphasizing one side of her personality, of her life - career, artistic talent, being a good mother, and so on. Sex is only a by-product of her life with him.

Important: *In spite of everything that has been said, the Aquarius woman reveals her claws good and proper when she discovers that her partner has been cheating on her!*

According to sextrology, the favorite positions of the Aquarius female are 1-1, 4-1, 12-3, 7-1 (not necessarily in that order).
For details, see the chapter on positions.

According to Western Astrology

The relationship between the Aquarius male/female and the members of the other signs:

Aries:
A spiritual relationship is favored over a physical one.

Taurus:
Disputes.

Gemini:
Married in spirit, but unfaithful in body.

Cancer:
Differences of opinion in spiritual and physical matters.

Leo:
Mutual admiration overcomes any obstacle.

Virgo:
A little in common, many differences.

Libra:
A happy couple.

Scorpio:
Opposing aims are not beneficial.

According to Western Astrology

Sagittarius:
A happy love affair - but not such a happy marriage.

Capricorn:
A rare relationship.

Aquarius:
A full life.

Pisces:
They both feel that they've missed out on something in life - and look elsewhere.

Sextrology

The aim of this questionnaire is to determine how well the **Aquarius man** matches the sextrological profile presented in this book.

Answer only Yes or No for each question. It is mandatory to answer all the questions.

Yes/No 1. Do you believe that in sex there are areas and boundaries that are "permitted" and "prohibited"?

Yes/No 2. Is it true that you don't go in for sexual variations and prefer the safe and known to the bizarre and mysterious?

Yes/No 3. Do you believe that sex is something that is done at night in bed?

Yes/No 4. Do you sometimes find yourself avoiding sex by using "feminine" excuses (such as a headache, etc.)?

Yes/No 5. In a relationship, do you adopt a certain sexual style from which you do not deviate?

Yes/No 6. Do you consider sex more of a duty than a pleasure?

Yes/No 7. Do you think you can bloom sexually only with a loving, understanding and faithful partner?

Add up the positive answers.

If you answered "Yes" to one or two of the questions, you match the profile of the Aquarius man "poorly."

If you answered "Yes" to three, four, or five of the questions, you match the profile of the Aquarius man "in an average and normal way."

If you answered "Yes" to six or seven of the questions, you match the profile of the Aquarius man "well."

Sextrology

Now we will add the questionnaire that the expert in Indian astrology and in the *Kama Sutra* would have constructed:

Do you define yourself as a rabbit, an ox, or a horse?

Now find the category to which you belong by following the simple procedure below:

(1) Circle the category (Rabbit, Ox, or Horse) that describes you.

(2) Circle the category (Poorly, Average & normal, or Well) according to your questionnaire score.

(3) Find the number where the two above categories meet. This number is your sextrological matching number.

	Rabbit	**Ox**	**Horse**
Poorly	1	2	3
Average & normal	4	5	6
Well	7	8	9

Sextrology

The aim of this questionnaire is to determine how well the **Aquarius woman** matches the sextrological profile presented in

Answer only Yes or No for each question. It is mandatory to answer all the questions.

Yes/No 1. You know that there are women who are more beautiful, richer, and smarter than you - but do you believe that you are the best when it comes to sexuality?

Yes/No 2. Is it true that you mainly - and sometimes only - like sex when you and your partner do what you like to do?

Yes/No 3. Is it true that you do not feel comfortable in a relationship with a man who used to be with one of your friends?

Yes/No 4. Is it true that you would never think of your partner as inferior to you?

Yes/No 5. Is it true that you would never allow your partner to tie up your hands and feet during sex?

Yes/No 6. Are you certain that if your partner raises a hand to you, it will be the end of your relationship?

Yes/No 7. Do you remember every particularly successful act of lovemaking that you ever experienced?

Add up the positive answers.

If you answered "Yes" to one or two of the questions, you match the profile of the Aquarius woman "poorly."

If you answered "Yes" to three, four, or five of the questions, you match the profile of the Aquarius woman "in an average and normal way."

Sextrology

If you answered "Yes" to six or seven of the questions, you match the profile of the Aquarius woman "well."

Now we will add the questionnaire that the expert in Indian astrology and in the *Kama Sutra* would have constructed:

Do you define yourself as a deer, a mare, or an elephant?

Now find the category to which you belong by following the simple procedure below:

(1) Circle the category (Deer, Mare, or Elephant) that describes you.
(2) Circle the category (Poorly, Average & normal, or Well) according to you questionnaire score.
(3) Find the number where the two above categories meet. This number is your sextrological matching number.

	Deer	**Mare**	**Elephant**
Poor	1	2	3
Average & normal	4	5	6
Well	7	8	9

According to Western Astrology

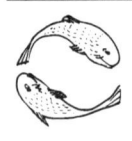

Pisces

Pisces people are idealists who do not always distinguish between dream and reality. They are the greatest romantics who sink into great loves, fall in love with glamorous movie stars and knights on white steeds, and whose hearts are broken every time their dreams are shattered by reality. The connection that Pisces people - males and females alike - make between "the great love" and reality leads to a large gap in expectations further along the line. Pisces females are disappointed to discover that the prince of their dreams is like any other man, and Pisces males wise up when they realize that their wonderful dreams are flesh and blood, just like they are.

Pisces people get married quite young, and direct their dreams of princes and princesses toward their children. They always hope that their children will be granted the happiness they themselves dreamed of in their childhood.

The romantic period in Pisces people's lives is quite short, and in the second part of their lives they are already saturated with disillusionment. Everyday life takes the place of moonlight strolls.

Although Pisces males are not always passionate lovers, they are full of love and pleasure, and an understanding partner can use this quality for her enjoyment.

In many cases, Pisces females are loving women, although their love is more spiritual than physical.

The Pisces male

The Pisces male belongs to the very last sign of the Zodiac.

Unlike what his name suggests, he is warm and loving, and is a powerful and considerate lover.

The Pisces male cannot separate sex from his love for his partner, and this is his virtue. He gives himself entirely, body and penis, to his partner.

Sometimes, during intercourse, it seems as if he is attached to his penis, rather than his penis being attached to him.

He will be amenable to any request his partner might make, and loves any position that she loves.

His penis is not big, his body is not muscular, and he is not wonderfully handsome, but the Pisces male is known as a lady-killer (although he doesn't "kill" too many of them!).

He is faithful and stable, and after a few sessions with a partner, he knows her well, and is adept at making his way around her depths.

Like the fish, which lives in water, seeks stability, so the Pisces male feels uncomfortable with a casual partner - so much so that sometimes his water element overwhelms his earth element, and his penis just won't oblige. This "glitch" does not happen to the Pisces male with his regular partner.

Sextrology

Important: *As in an aquarium, the Pisces male also needs clean water in order to ensure the flow of oxygen. Don't try to repress him, otherwise he will dehydrate.*

According to sextrology, the favorite positions of the Pisces male are 5-2, 8-3, 6-3, 10-2 (not necessarily in that order).
For details, see the chapter on positions.

The Pisces female

The Pisces female is the ideal woman from the romantic novels... she falls in love, she follows her love, she is attracted to his charms... but she does not make love with him between the pages of the book!

For the Pisces female, a kiss is a true sexual adventure. What a shame. She has real sexual potential, but it is difficult to expose and fulfill it. There are many Pisces females for whom only giving birth releases the spring of sexuality.

The Pisces female falls in love easily, surrenders to every bouquet of flowers and box of candies, melts when receiving a compliment... and defends her virginity against every assault!

Sometimes, even though she reaches the stage of kissing and caressing, she keeps her private parts as tightly sealed as a bank vault. It is not rare to find Pisces females who are still virgins after long months of marriage!

A long time - and the right man - are required to extricate the Pisces female from her romantic fantasies and get her into the world of the senses. And not every man has the patience for this undertaking.

The Pisces female can, of course, take herself in hand, change her character, and realize her romantic fantasies between the sheets... but that depends entirely on her!

Sextrology

The change must stem from her own decision, and not from outside influences.

Important: *During pregnancy and for a long time after giving birth, the Pisces female will stay away from sex as if it were a disease. That's a real shame!*

According to sextrology, the favorite positions of the Pisces female are 4-3, 1-2, 8-3, 3-2 (not necessarily in that order).
For details, see the chapter on positions.

According to Western Astrology

The relationship between the Pisces male/female and the members of the other signs:

Aries:
Tension and anxiety are detrimental to pleasure.

Taurus:
A match that fulfills itself.

Gemini:
Mutual pursuit of pleasures.

Cancer:
A relationship in which "a little contains a lot."

Leo:
Contradictory aims are not beneficial.

Virgo:
A relationship that does not work very often.

Libra:
A happy couple.

Scorpio:
A relationship that is more spiritual than physical.

According to Western Astrology

Sagittarius:
Romance, which is not often expressed physically.

Capricorn:
Complete fulfillment.

Aquarius:
Their eyes are too big! They want everything but only get a little.

Pisces:
A happy couple in everyday life.

Sextrology

The aim of this questionnaire is to determine how well the **Pisces man** matches the sextrological profile presented in this book.

Answer only Yes or No for each question. It is mandatory to answer all the questions.

Yes/No 1. Do you believe that sexual technique and experience are preferable to unbridled emotion and lust?

Yes/No 2. Do you believe that a man must experience a wide variety of sex?

Yes/No 3. Is it true that while you don't particularly believe in fidelity, you aren't jealous or possessive?

Yes/No 4. Is it true that you can be the perfect lover with the right partner at the right time... if you want?

Yes/No 5. Do you aspire to be a lover who is different than all your partner's previous lovers (and the emphasis here is on different, not better)?

Yes/No 6. Are you prepared to "try" anything, at least once?

Yes/No 7. Is it true that your partner's pleasure is just as important to you as your own?

Add up the positive answers.

If you answered "Yes" to one or two of the questions, you match the profile of the Pisces man "poorly."

If you answered "Yes" to three, four, or five of the questions, you match the profile of the Pisces man "in an average and normal way."

If you answered "Yes" to six or seven of the questions, you match the profile of the Pisces man "well."

Sextrology

Now we will add the questionnaire that the expert in Indian astrology and in the *Kama Sutra* would have constructed:

Do you define yourself as a rabbit, an ox, or a horse?

Now find the category to which you belong by following the simple procedure below:

(1) Circle the category (Rabbit, Ox, or Horse) that describes you.

(2) Circle the category (Poorly, Average & normal, or Well) according to your questionnaire score.

(3) Find the number where the two above categories meet. This number is your sextrological matching number.

	Rabbit	**Ox**	**Horse**
Poorly	1	2	3
Average & normal	4	5	6
Well	7	8	9

Sextrology

The aim of this questionnaire is to determine how well the **Pisces woman** matches the sextrological profile presented in this book.

Answer only Yes or No for each question. It is mandatory to answer all the questions.

Yes/No 1. Do you believe that sex "binds" your partner to you?
Yes/No 2. Do you believe that a woman has to adapt herself to her husband's sexual desires?
Yes/No 3. Do you believe that romance is the best way to achieve orgasm?
Yes/No 4. Are you always prepared to watch an erotic movie in the presence of other people?
Yes/No 5. When you feel depressed, upset, or hurt, can sex improve your mood?
Yes/No 6. Is it true that dirty language cools your desire and prevents you from reaching orgasm?
Yes/No 7. Is it true that you sometimes describe your partner as perfect in every way, a veritable knight on a white steed (for you)?

Add up the positive answers.

If you answered "Yes" to one or two of the questions, you match the profile of the Pisces woman "poorly."

If you answered "Yes" to three, four, or five of the questions, you match the profile of the Pisces woman "in an average and normal way."

If you answered "Yes" to six or seven of the questions, you match the profile of the Pisces woman "well."

Sextrology

Now we will add the questionnaire that the expert in Indian astrology and in the *Kama Sutra* would have constructed:

Do you define yourself as a deer, a mare, or an elephant?

Now find the category to which you belong by following the simple procedure below:

(1) Circle the category (Deer, Mare, or Elephant) that describes you.

(2) Circle the category (Poorly, Average & normal, or Well) according to you questionnaire score.

(3) Find the number where the two above categories meet. This number is your sextrological matching number.

	Deer	**Mare**	**Elephant**
Poor	1	2	3
Average & normal	4	5	6
Well	7	8	9